Communications
in Computer and Information Science   464

More information about this series at http://www.springer.com/series/7899

Jan Cabri · Pedro Pezarat Correia
João Barreiros (Eds.)

Sports Science Research and Technology Support

International Congress, icSPORTS 2013
Vilamoura, Algarve, Portugal,
September 20–22, 2013
Revised Selected Papers

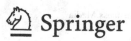
Springer

Editors
Jan Cabri
Norwegian School of Sport Sciences
Oslo
Norway

João Barreiros
University of Lisbon
Cruz Quebrada
Portugal

Pedro Pezarat Correia
University of Lisbon
Cruz Quebrada
Portugal

ISSN 1865-0929   ISSN 1865-0937 (electronic)
Communications in Computer and Information Science
ISBN 978-3-319-17547-8   ISBN 978-3-319-17548-5 (eBook)
DOI 10.1007/978-3-319-17548-5

Library of Congress Control Number: 2015937496

Springer Cham Heidelberg New York Dordrecht London

Printed on acid-free paper

Springer International Publishing AG Switzerland is part of Springer Science+Business Media
(www.springer.com)

Preface

The present book includes extended and revised versions of a set of selected papers from the First International Congress on Sport Science Research and Technology Support (icSPORTS 2013), held in Vilamoura, Algarve, Portugal from 20 to 22 September, 2013.

The purpose of the International Congress on Sport Science Research and Technology Support is to bring together researchers and practitioners in order to exchange ideas and develop synergies highlighting the benefits of any kind of technology for sports either in general of regarding a particular case of application.

icSPORTS 2013 was co-sponsored by INSTICC (Institute for Systems and Technologies of Information, Control, and Communication) and SportTools, Technology for Sport. icSPORTS has the institutional sponsorship of the University of Lisbon, the Norwegian School of Sport Sciences, the Olympic Committee of Portugal; Portuguese Golf Federation; Portuguese Surf Federation; Portuguese Institute of Sports and Youth and Portuguese Federation of Sports for Disabled. icSPORTS. It was held in cooperation with the European College of Sport Science (ECSS); European College of Sports and Exercise Physicians (ECOSEP); Sociedade Portuguesa de Biomecânica (SPB), BenficaLab, Portuguese Society of Physioterapists (APF), and technically co-sponsored by the International Association of Computer Science in Sport (IACSS).

The congress received 90 paper submissions from 32 countries in all continents. To evaluate each submission, a double-blind paper review was performed by the Program Committee. After a stringent selection process, papers were published and presented as full papers, i.e., completed work (30' oral presentation), leading to a "full-paper" acceptance ratio of about 16 %, which shows the intention of preserving a high-quality forum for the next editions of this congress.

icSPORTS's program included panels and four invited talks delivered by internationally distinguished speakers, namely: James S. Skinner (Indiana University, United States); Marco Narici (University of Nottingham, United Kingdom); Robert J. Neal, (Golf BioDynamics, United States) and François Hug (University of Queensland, Australia).

We would like to thank the authors, whose research and development efforts are recorded here for future generations.

October 2014

Jan Cabri
João Barreiros
Pedro Pezarat Correia

Organization

Congress Chair

Jan Cabri   Norwegian School of Sport Sciences, Norway

Program Co-chairs

Pedro Pezarat Correia   University of Lisbon, Portugal
João Barreiros   University of Lisbon, Portugal

Organizing Committee

Marina Carvalho   INSTICC, Portugal
Helder Coelhas   INSTICC, Portugal
Bruno Encarnação   INSTICC, Portugal
Ana Guerreiro   INSTICC, Portugal
André Lista   INSTICC, Portugal
Andreia Moita   INSTICC, Portugal
Raquel Pedrosa   INSTICC, Portugal
Vitor Pedrosa   INSTICC, Portugal
Cláudia Pinto   INSTICC, Portugal
Susana Ribeiro   INSTICC, Portugal
Sara Santiago   INSTICC, Portugal
Mara Silva   INSTICC, Portugal
José Varela   INSTICC, Portugal
Pedro Varela   INSTICC, Portugal

Program Committee

María Ángeles Pérez Ansón   University of Zaragoza, Spain
Duarte Araújo   Faculdade de Motricidade Humana - Universidade
                             de Lisboa, Portugal
Arnold Baca   University of Vienna, Austria
Marco Barbero   University of Applied Sciences and Arts
                             of Southern Switzerland, Switzerland
José Angelo Barela   Universidade Cruzeiro do Sul, Brazil
Mickael Begon   Université de Montréal, Canada
Rodrigo Rico Bini   Universidade Federal do Rio Grande do Sul, Brazil
David Bishop   Victoria University, Australia
Maarten Bobbert   VU University in Amsterdam, The Netherlands
Daniel Boullosa   Universidade Católica de Brasília, Brazil

Mark King	Loughborough University, UK
Andrey Koptyug	Mid Sweden University, Sweden
Nicola Lai	Case Western Reserve University, USA
Anthony Leicht	James Cook University, Australia
Silvio lorenzetti	Institute for Biomechanics, ETH Zurich, Switzerland
Ric Lovell	The University of Western Sydney, UK
Keith Lyons	University of Canberra, Australia
Kelly Mackintosh	Swansea University, UK
Sean Maw	Mount Royal University, Canada
Melitta McNarry	Swansea University, UK
Alberto Mendes-Villanueva	ASPIRE Academy of Sports Excellence, Qatar
Amir Ali Mohagheghi	Brunel University London, UK
Geraldine Naughton	Australian Catholic University, Australia
Raúl Oliveira	Faculdade de Motricidade Humana - Universidade de Lisboa, Portugal
Matthew Pain	Loughborough University, UK
Pedro Passos	Faculdade de Motricidade Humana - Universidade de Lisboa, Portugal
Noel Perkins	University of Michigan, USA
Alessandro Pezzoli	Politecnico di Torino - University of Turin, Italy
Mary Rodgers	University of Maryland, USA
Scott Sailor	California State University, Fresno, USA
James S. Skinner	Indiana University, USA
Christos Spitas	Delft University of Technology, The Netherlands
Ben Stansfield	Glasgow Caledonian University, UK
Kazumoto Tanaka	Kinki University, Japan
David Thiel	Griffith University, Australia
Herbert Ugrinowitsch	Universidade Federal de Minas Gerais, Brazil
Kirsti Uusi-Rasi	UKK Institute for Health Promotion Research, Finland
Benedicte Vanwanseele	Catholic University Leuven, Belgium
Evert Verhagen	VU University Amsterdam, University Medical Centre, The Netherlands
Hans Weghorn	BW Cooperative State University Stuttgart, Germany
Fabio Zaina	ISICO, Italy
Yanxin Zhang	The University of Auckland, New Zealand

Auxiliary Reviewers

| Marco Aguiar | University of Trás-os-Montes e Alto Douro, Portugal |
| Bruno Baroni | Federal University of Rio Grande do Sul, Brazil |

Pedro Silva   Faculdade de Desporto, Universidade de Porto,
                    Portugal
Bruno Travassos   University of Beira Interior, Portugal

Invited Speakers

James S. Skinner   Indiana University, USA
Marco Narici   University of Nottingham, UK
Robert J. Neal   Golf BioDynamics, USA
François Hug   The University of Queensland, Australia

Contents

Contents

Effect of the Environment on the Sport Performance: Computer Supported Training - A Case Study for Cycling Sports

Alessandro Pezzoli[1,2(✉)], Elena Cristofori[1,2], Matteo Moncalero[2,3],
Fiorella Giacometto[2,4], Andrea Boscolo[2],
Roberto Bellasio[5], and Jacopo Padoan[6]

[1] DIST, Politecnico di Torino - Università di Torino, Turin, Italy
{alessandro.pezzoli,elena.cristofori}@polito.it
[2] R.U. MeteoSport, DIST, Politecnico di Torino - Università di Torino,
Turin, Italy
andrea.b@atleticom.it
fiorella.giacometto@libero.it
[3] DICAM, Alma Mater Studiorum, Università di Bologna, Bologna, Italy
matteo.moncalero@unibo.it
[4] Ospedale Cottolengo, Piccola Casa della Divina Provvidenza, Turin, Italy
[5] Enviroware, Concorezzo, Monza-Brianza, Italy
rbellasio@enviroware.com
[6] FLJ Sport Solution, Turin, Italy
jacopo.padoan@alice.it

Abstract. The effect of weather and environmental conditions on sports has been extensively studied over the last few years. Most of the outdoor sport activities, and in particular endurance sports, are strongly influenced by the variation of meteorological parameters.

Notwithstanding the conditions of the outdoor environment are often not considered when evaluating sport performances, as if they were not important, the sport performances are strongly related to the environmental conditions.

The aim of this paper is to assess how much atmospheric variables may influence both the athletic performance and the comfort level for different sport disciplines. The analysis of a case study, focused on the cycling sport, shows how the computer supported training can help the Coaches and the Athletes to consider simultaneously the sport performance and the environmental data.

Keywords: Sport performance · Environmental data · Computer supported training · Cycling

1 Introduction

Environmental and meteorological conditions have an important effect on outdoor sport performances. For instance wind direction and wind speed are important, during marathons, rowing and sailing races [1]. Air temperature is also very important during long running events.

© Springer International Publishing Switzerland 2015
J. Cabri et al. (Eds.): icSPORTS 2013, CCIS 464, pp. 1–16, 2015.
DOI: 10.1007/978-3-319-17548-5_1

Considering marathons, the American College of Sports Medicine has established guidelines for preventing health effects due to extreme weather conditions [2]. The guidelines are based on the "wet bulb-globe-temperature" index (WBGT index) which is based on the combined effects of air temperature, relative humidity, radiant heat and air movement. For example race cancellation or voluntary withdrawal are recommended when WBGT > 28 °C. Recently El Helou et al. [3] found that air temperature and performance are significantly correlated.

In effect the assessment of bio-climatological conditions and of thermal comfort in endurance sports, particularly in road cycling, is essential not only for a proper planning of the training program and the nutritional plan, but also for a better evaluation of the racing strategy [4, 5].

Water temperature, for example, plays an important role in swimming, particularly during triathlon races. Indeed, below 13 °C, the maximum swim distance is usually shortened (e.g. Rulebook of the British Triathlon Federation). Moreover, at temperatures below 11 °C it is recommended that open water swimming does not take place.

Among the meteorological variables that strongly influence the sport activity the most important are temperature, wind, precipitation, fog, atmospheric pressure and relative humidity. The usefulness of weather forecasts in performance sports management has been demonstrated by Pezzoli et al. [5] and Pezzoli and Cristofori [6]. The results obtained by such Authors show how the role of the meteorological parameters becomes crucial for sporting activities carried out in an outdoor environment.

Beside meteorological variables, other environmental variables play an important role, such as, for example, pollution levels. It is well known and demonstrated [7, 8] that the air concentration of particulate matter (PM10 and PM2.5) has deleterious effects on the respiratory functions, even if they persist only for short times. The same statement holds for other pollutants.

Notwithstanding the conditions of the outdoor environment are often not considered when evaluating sport performances, as if they were not important, the sport performances are strongly related to the environmental conditions [9].

The aim of this paper is to assess how much atmospheric variables may influence both the athletic performance and the comfort level for different sport disciplines. The availability of these specific information leads to a more detailed knowledge of the race area and opens up the possibility of making considerations on past trends, as well as on the predictability of future atmospheric situations and meteorological phenomena.

This research is articulated in three parts. The first one is based on a new methodology that, by means of structured interviews to athletes and coaches of the major national teams of the Italian Olympic Committee, has shown how environmental variables may influence sport performances. Then it has been studied how different lead-time weather forecasts can contribute to the improvement of the performance itself.

In the second part is analyzed how, a specific software, which consider simultaneously environmental data and sport activity parameters, may help coaches and athletes to better evaluate their performance.

The third part of the research has been devoted to the analysis of a case study applied to the cycling sport. In this context, some tests carried out with the help of a professional athlete, have demonstrated the actual influence of the environmental parameters on the sport performance. The results confirm the need to develop a specific software capable of integrating simultaneously the analysis of sport activity parameters and the environmental data.

2 Methods and Materials

This paragraph analyzes the methods adopted and the materials used to develop the research, during the three different phases described above (environmental analysis, software for analyzing environmental data and sport performances, case study).

2.1 Environment and Sport Performance

Based on Lobozewicz [10], Kay and Vamplew [11] and Pezzoli and Cristofori [6] studies, it was conducted a qualitative-quantitative assessment of the influence of environmental variables on sport performance using the Haddon matrix [12].

William Haddon Jr. developed his conceptual model, the Haddon matrix, in 1980. Since that time, the matrix has been used as a tool to assist in developing ideas for preventing injuries of many types.

The application of the Haddon matrix in the field of the sports activities allows to determine the factors that mostly affect the performance, such as (Fig. 1):

- Personal factors (psychophysical preparation);
- Vector or Agent Factors (materials and opponent);
- Physical Environmental factors (meteorological and environmental analysis). Hereafter the "Physical Environmental factors" will be called "environmental parameters" and they will be referred to meteorological parameters (i.e.: air temperature, air humidity, wind, rain, etc....) that affect the sport performance;
- Socio-environmental factors (of internal and external social environment).

Focusing on Fig. 1, and in particular on the column "Physical – Environmental Factors", it is evident how different methodologies have to be used for the analysis of the environmental parameters during the different temporal phases of a specific sport event. During the pre-event phase a climatological and statistical analysis proves to be the most suitable. On the other hand, during the event, a deterministic forecast methodology, associated with very short-term numerical weather prediction models, is

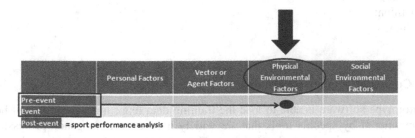

Fig. 1. Haddon matrix.

suggested. Finally, in the post-event phase meteorological measurements can be used, if available, for refining the performance analysis.

If the environmental parameters are not taken into account, one column would be missing within the Haddon matrix and hence an error would be produced using the performance assessment model.

The importance of Environmental Analysis for sport performance is often underestimated by coaches and sport managers. This is mostly due to the lack of knowledge about the added value brought by innovative techniques for both measuring and predicting environmental parameters.

The different time-scales for conducting a proper environmental analysis and a weather forecasting, during a general sport event, can be divided as follows:

- Long term (up to 30 days before the event);
- Medium term (from 30 days before the event to 8 days before the event);
- Short term (from 8 days to 6 h before the event);
- Very short term (from 6 h before the event until the 'action').

This subdivision, and the related weather forecasts, have to be used with regard to the possibilities offered by each Sports' Rule for what concerns the use of meteorological information.

With this kind of meteorological analysis, and according to the Haddon matrix, a proper assessment of the environmental parameter is assured.

A series of in-depth focus groups conducted with different stakeholders (athletes, coaches, managers, performance analysts) coming from the main National Sports Federations of the Italian Olympic Committee (CONI) has allowed to estimate the importance of meteorological variables and the impact of different lead-time weather forecasts on the general performance, for several sports [13, 14].

In particular the following disciplines have been analyzed:

- Cycling: road;
- Rowing;
- Canoe and Kayak;
- Athletics: Marathon and Race Walks;
- Modern Pentathlon;
- Equestrian Sports;
- Tennis;
- Archery;
- Shooting Sports;
- Triathlon;
- Sailing.

2.2   Computer Supported Training

The prototype software is able to load the training data (e.g.: time, position and heart rate) monitored by specific tools that are widely used even among non-professional practitioners (Garmin, Polar, Suunto, etc.). The software tool is also able to load the meteorological data, or other environmental data, measured by one or more monitoring stations of interest. Other important data to analyze are those monitored on the athlete, such as for example his/her skin temperature or humidity [5]. These last data are important when testing the features of particular clothing. All the above mentioned data are generally measured in different positions and in different times. In order to carry out the analysis all the external data must be time interpolated to get them on the same times at which the performance is available (synchronization process).

In a similar way, when the meteorological data are measured by more than one station, a spatial interpolation is needed to estimate the values at the same positions where the performance has been registered. There are situations where it is not correct to perform the spatial interpolation, in such cases it is possible to indicate a radius of influence of each station, or to define areas of competence of each monitoring stations.

Of course the spatial interpolation may be more reasonable in some situations than in other ones. For example, if N stations are measuring wind speed and direction during a sailing race over a relative small water surface, the spatial interpolation is more than reasonable. On the other hand, if the same number of stations is measuring the same variables during a cycling race over a mountain region, the simple spatial interpolation might not be reasonable. In such cases a diagnostic meteorological model (e.g. CALMET) would do a better work, but it cannot be easily incorporated in a software as the one described here.

For other variables, such as temperature, specific algorithms are available to carry out spatial interpolation even in complex terrain [15]. Indeed, air temperature at the ground depends on some variables, such as altitude above sea level, air temperature vertical gradient and land cover type. The interpolation of sparse measurements of temperature over the domain should account for these parameters.

Other meteorological variables are calculated by the software if not available among the measurements. For example, solar radiation can be estimated starting from the geographic location of the athlete, which depends on the time, and on cloud cover, which can be obtained, for example, from METAR (Meteorological Aerodrome Report) data.

The software is developed with .NET framework 3.5 in Visual Basic language. The cartographic layers has to be found by an Open Access map to be used freely by the Coaches and the Athletes. The Open Street map [16] is an efficient GIS data that can be integrated into the sports performance software.

2.3 Case Study: Cycling

Considering the contents of the two previous paragraphs, it has been decided to apply the environmental analysis to a sport which is particularly influenced by the environmental conditions. For these reasons the sport of cycling has been chosen since, as it will be shown later in this paper, it is strongly influenced both by environmental conditions and by weather conditions.

In order to carry out the tests, whose results have been analyzed with the computerized methodology described in Sect. 2.2, the protocol developed by Pezzoli et al. [5] has been applied. Particular attention has been given to the following topics:

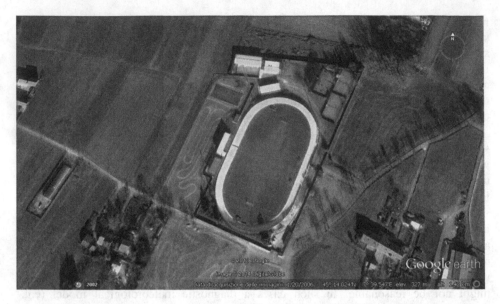

Fig. 2. Track of San Francesco al Campo, Turin – Piedmont – Italy.

- Study of the test course. It has been decided to carry out the tests on an oval track, in order to keep constant some important variables (altitude, slope, etc.) and to avoid the introduction of possible bias factors. In this way the repeatability of the test conditions has been guaranteed, making comparable the results obtained in the different test sessions. The tests have been carried out on the circuit of San Francesco al Campo, Turin, Piedmont, Italy (Fig. 2).
- Environmental analysis of the race course. The tests took place on 2 September 2013, from 10:25 LT to 11:55 LT, and all the environmental parameters have been measured during this time interval. The following meteorological variables have been measured in continuous with a sampling rate of 1':

    (a) Wind direction and speed;
    (b) Air temperature;
    (c) Relative humidity;
    (d) Atmospheric pressure.

An high-precision anemometer (JDC – SKYWATCH Geos 11) was used; this tool has already proved extremely performing in the application of meteorology to sport [5]. The meteorological variables have been used to calculate the apparent temperature index. Considering the studies of Leung et al. [17] and Robaa [18] it has been decided to use the NET index, which is more complete of the Heat Index (HI) and of the Windchill (WC) because it is also a function of wind speed, in addition to air temperature and relative humidity.

Finally the temperature of the track surface has been measured in continuous with a sampling time of 15″ by means of a thermocouple recording thermometer model JDC - Center 306.

- Research of a target athlete and of clothing for the test. It has been decided to work with a single professional athlete, belonging to a high-level elite, capable to guarantee the perfect reproducibility of the tests. Two different typologies of clothing have been compared in order to verify that the described protocol, and the software, are capable to give reliable results with respect to the expected results:

  (a) "Infrared Carbon" short-sleeved shirt and shorts, manufactured by B-Emme;
  (b) Ceramic short-sleeved shirt and shorts, manufactured by B-Emme.

- Performance analysis. The aim of this analysis is to detect the different values of power expressed by athletes in different test conditions and consequently to evaluate the internal heat production expressed in Watt (W). During this phase the following parameters have been constantly registered: power, speed, cadence of pedaling, slope of the road and heart rate. The power and the related internal heat production have been measured using the PowerTap system. To measure the skin temperature, it was decided to use the iButtons, small sensors constituted by a chip enclosed in stainless steel which is 16 mm thick (Fig. 3). Due to its very small size, the instrument can be easily applied to the skin of the tester without interfering with the movement or the technical gesture. The iButton can be mounted virtually anywhere because it is rugged enough to withstand harsh environments (indoors or outdoors). It has many application fields, lately it has also been used in different sports for the measurement of environmental parameters [19]. Six iButtons have been used, placed in pairs on the right and on the left of the following muscles: pectorals, lumbar, and dorsal.

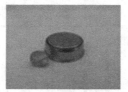

Fig. 3. iButton.

- Test protocol. A total of five tests has been carried out. The first one, appositely performed to bring the tester to a regime situation, has been discarded because the athlete did not reach the sweating condition. Then two pairs of tests have been performed changing the two previously-described types of clothing. The two intermediate tests (i.e. tests 2 and 3) have been analyzed. Tests 4 and 5 were still significant, however it has been preferred not to use them because the athlete already did three tests reaching the threshold conditions. The tests have been done according to the following protocol:

  (a) 3′ of "dead time" to entry and exit from the plant;
  (b) 4′ at average-frequency intensity (250–290 W);
  (c) 3′ at threshold intensity (320–380 W).

3 Results

The results of the research are analyzed in the following parts, considering the three different phases (environmental analysis, software for analyzing environmental data and sport performances, case study).

3.1 Environment and Sport Performance

The analysis of the data extracted from the focus groups, showed that each of the analyzed sports is strongly influenced by the following meteorological variables:

- Temperature;
- Humidity;
- Wind.

Some sports, and among them tennis, cycling and, in general, all shooting disciplines, are also influenced by rain and fog (Fig. 4).

It was also observed the high impact that long-term weather forecasting can have on all sports considered (Fig. 4). This analysis leads to believe that all major sporting events (Olympics, World Championships) are to be considered as "situ-specific". Then athletes, coaches and technicians can use a careful climatological analysis to finalize the sports training well in advance from the date of the event.

		Impact of meteorological parameters on the sport performance						Impact of the meteorological forecast at different time-scales on the sport performance			
Sport	Disciplines	Atmospheric Pressure	Air Temperature	Wind	Rain	Fog	Air Humidity	Long term (up to 30 days before the event)	Medium term (from 30 days before the event to 8 days before the event)	Short term (from 8 days to 6 hours before the event)	Very short term (from 6 hours before the event until the 'action')
Cycling	road	3	4	5	4	3	4	5	4	3	2
Rowing	all	2	4	5	3	1	4	5	5	4	4
noe & kayak	all	2	4	5	3	1	4	5	4	3	2
Athletics	Marathon - Race Walks	2	5	3	3	3	5	5	5	3	1
Modern Pentathlon	Equitation, Running, Shooting	2	5	5	3	5	5	5	4	3	3
Equestrian Sports	all	1	5	3	3	4	5	5	5	4	3
Tennis	all	1	4	4	5	5	4	5	4	3	1
Archery	all	1	3	5	3	4	3	5	4	4	5
Shooting Sports	all	1	2	5	4	5	2	5	4	4	3
Triathlon	all	3	4	5	4	2	4	5	4	4	2
Sailing	all	1	4	5	3	4	4	5	5	5	5

Impact Index: 1 = Very Low; 2 = Low; 3 = Medium; 4 = High; 5 = Very high

Fig. 4. Impact of meteorological parameters and meteorological forecast on the sport performance.

		Weather forecast at different time scale and impact on the improving of the sports performance			
Sport	Disciplines	Long term (up to 30 days before the event)	Medium term (from 30 days before the event to 8 days before the event)	Short term (from 8 days to 6 hours before the event)	Very short term (from 6 hours before the event until the 'action')
Cycling	road	training program (physical and mental); decision about the training's site; nutrition planning; material development	training program (physical and mental); nutrition planning (hydration); strategy of the race	nutrition planning (hydration); mental training; pre-race conditioning; selection of the bicycle and clothing; strategy of the race; decision of the placement on the bike	nutrition planning (hydration); strategy of the race
Rowing	all	training program (physical and mental); decision about the training's site; nutrition planning; material development	training program (physical and mental); nutrition planning (hydration); trim of the boat	nutrition planning (hydration); mental training; pre-race conditioning; selection of material; strategy of the race; post-race conditioning	trim of the boat

Fig. 5. Impact of weather forecast at different time scale on the improving of the sport performance (example for cycling and rowing).

Finally, it was evaluated as the weather forecast with different lead-times can be used to improve sports performance (Fig. 5).

This further analysis confirms that the sports training of an athlete should be considered as a complex system where only the correct interaction between information from different sources can lead to the achievement of excellence's performance.

3.2 Computer Supported Training

The software reproduces the training track on a map (the Open Street Map database is used), and for each point a lot of information is given as, for example, wind speed and direction in a specific training location, temperature, or important indices such as the wind chill or the Net Effective Temperature [17]. Of course, each point is also related to the training data, as for example, the time elapsed from the start of the exercise, the total distance, the average and instantaneous speeds, the heart rate, etc. The user is also allowed to export the track in KML or KMZ format in order to view it on Google Earth.

The performances are also summarized in tabular format, and the user is allowed to export the tables in many formats in order to use them in presentations or for further analysis.

The first version of the software is still being developed as a desktop application for PCs. Future versions could be available also for Android and iOS tablets.

The basic idea of the development of the software are reviewed in Fig. 6.

As shown by Fig. 6 an important part of the software is related to the time and space interpolation. By means of the methodology described by Bellasio et al. [15] it is possible to interpolate the surface temperature at any point of the domain considering also the terrain elevation of the meteorological stations and the type of surface by means of the leaf area index.

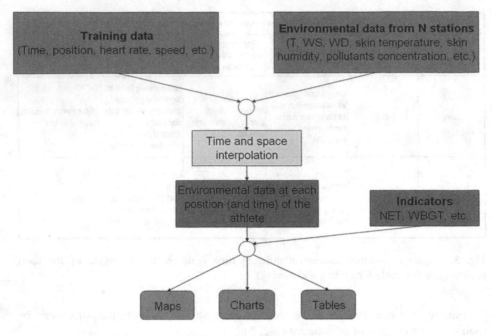

Fig. 6. Flow chart of the software.

All the measured and derived data (both referring to the sport performance and to the environment) will be represented in a synchronous way, by allowing coaches and athletes to analyze their performance to the light of the meteorological and environmental conditions at the time of the performance itself.

As it will be shown in the next paragraph, this kind of software is of great importance for the final user, since it allows to correctly consider all the parameters which influence the sport performance.

On the other hand, as illustrated in Sect. 3.1, it is no more possible to disregard the effects of environmental and meteorological parameters, as they greatly affect all the outdoor sports activities.

3.3   Case Study: Cycling

The computerized analysis of the meteorological and environmental data measured during the test (late morning of 2 September 2013) is summarized in Table 1.

Figure 7 shows the sport performance parameters monitored during the five tests. As shown in Table 2, during tests 2 and 3 the tester had physiological characteristics and speeds completely comparable, confirming the high reliability of the tester and, as a consequence, of the tests themselves.

Finally, two different sport clothing have been tested. According to the clothing manufacturer one should expect better results in test 3 than in test 2. In fact, the ceramic

Table 1. Environmental and meteorological data measured during the test.

Environmental Data	02-Sept-13
Test Hours	[10.25LT ; 11.55LT]
Apparent Temperature – Average [°C]	24.7
Apparent Temperature – Range 60% [°C]	[+23.0 ; +26.5]
Surface Track Temperature – Average [°C]	34.6
Surface Track Temperature – Range 60% [°C]	[+32.0 ; +37.1]
Sky	Clear

Table 2. Performance data. The square brackets indicate the 60 % of frequency of occurrence.

	Power [W]	Bike Speed [km/h]	Heart rate frequencies [bpm]
Test 2	282 [265;299]	39,6 [37.2;42]	158 [149;167]
Test 3	290 [273;307]	40 [37.5;42.5]	157 [148;166]

material has shown better transpiration features with respect to the "Infrared Carbon" material.

As shown by Figs. 8 and 9 and by Tables 3 and 4, prepared with the help of the integrated analysis software, at the moment of maximum effort the use of the ceramic material not only shows a drop in temperature in the breastplate, but also shows a sharp drop in humidity thanks to the "pumping" effect.

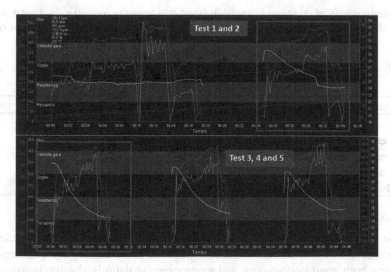

Fig. 7. Performance parameters: bike speed (blue line), heart rate (red line) and power (yellow line). The two tests considered for the analysis (tests 2 and 3) are reported within the red boxes (Color figure online).

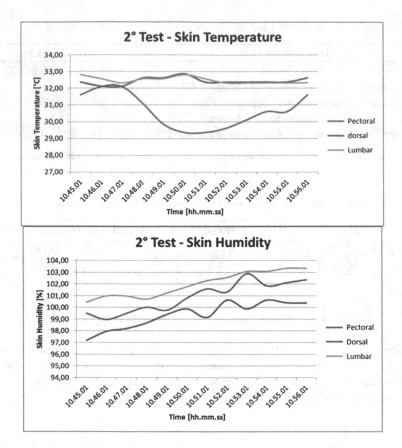

Fig. 8. Measurements of skin temperature (above) and skin humidity (below) carried out during test 2 ("Infrared Carbon" short-sleeved shirt and shorts, manufactured by B-Emme) (Color figure online).

Table 3. Data measured during the 2nd test.

Thermal Comfort Data	2nd Test
Hours	[10.45LT ; 10.56LT]
Skin Temperature – Average [°C]	31.8
Skin Temperature – Range [°C]	[31.4 ; 32.1]
Skin Humidity – Average [%]	100.6
Skin Humidity – Range [%]	[99.5 ; 101.7]

These tests show that, independently from the significance of the data obtained, a data processing tool that enables the user to analyze in synchrony all measured data (concerning both sport performance and environmental data) is absolutely essential.

All the analysis carried out with this kind of software can integrate in a holistic view the parameters that affect performance in sport.

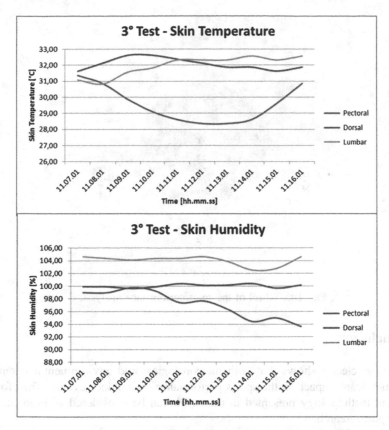

Fig. 9. Measurements of skin temperature (above) and skin humidity (below) carried out during test 2 (Ceramic short-sleeved shirt and shorts, manufactured by B-Emme) (Color figure online).

Table 4. Data measured during the 3rd test.

Thermal Comfort Data	3rd Test
Hours	[11.07LT ; 11.16LT]
Skin Temperature – Average [°C]	31.1
Skin Temperature – Range [°C]	[30.8 ; 31.4]
Skin Humidity – Average [%]	99.9
Skin Humidity – Range [%]	[99.0 ; 100.8]

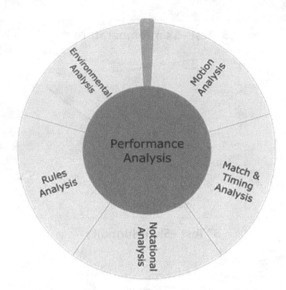

Fig. 10. Wheel of the sport performance analysis.

4 Conclusion

This analysis clearly shows that both meteorological and environmental parameters have a significant impact on the sports performance for outdoor events. Therefore the assessment methodology presented in this work can be considered as innovative for applied sport research.

It follows that the Performance Analyst should develop relevant competences needed for conducting an integrated data analysis, taking into account the environmental parameters as well.

Moreover the Performance Analyst has to take care of the results' communication of this integrated performance data analysis to the coaches through understandable and meaningful messages.

From the focus groups and from the case study, it was concluded that, in the sports Performance Analysis the following well-known areas need to be addressed (Fig. 10):

- Motion Analysis
- Match and Timing Analysis
- Notational Analysis

In addition to these areas, two new areas must be faced, namely:

- Rule Analysis
- Environmental Analysis

These considerations are in agreement with innovative researches carried out on the Team Sport [20–22], on the cycling [5], on the water sport [1] as well as in the winter sports [23, 24].

Therefore National Sports Federation should pay particular attention to train these specific competencies in order to create sports operators that can fulfill the role of Performance Analysts with the necessary awareness. In addition the technicians will need a specific and continuous education allowing the achievement of the fundamental knowledge in the field of environmental analysis.

Finally it has been demonstrated that the use of an innovative computer supported training system, taking into account all the sport performance parameters and the environmental conditions, can be useful for both coaches and athletes.

This tool, not yet developed in the Sport Technology, is able to deliver to both coaches and athletes added value information since it is simultaneously taking into account both the environmental and the sport performance values.

This technology that allows the comparison of the sport performance in relationship with the environmental conditions in which it was carried out, represents an innovative topic, within the 'environmental sensible' sports, which would need further investigations.

References

1. Pezzoli, A., Baldacci, A., Cama, A., Faina, M., DallaVedova, D., Besi, M., Vercelli, G., Boscolo, A., Moncalero, M., Cristofori, E., Dalessandro, M.: Wind-wave interactions in enclosed basins: the impact on the sport of rowing. In: Clanet, C. (ed.) Sport Physics, pp. 139–151. Ecole Polytechnique de Paris, Paris (2013)
2. Cantu, R.C., Micheli, L.J.: ACSM Guidelines for the Team Physician. Lea & Febiger Editors, Philadelphia (1991)
3. El Helou, N., Tafflet, M., Berthelot, G., Tolaini, J., Marc, A., Guillame, M., Hausswirth, C., Toussaint, J.F.: Impact of environmental parameters on marathon running performance. PLoS One 7(5), e37407 (2012)
4. Olds, T.S., Norton, K.I., Lowe, E.L., Olive, S., Reay, F., Ly, S.: Modelling road-cycling performance. J. Appl. Physiol. 78(4), 1596–1611 (1995)
5. Pezzoli, A., Cristofori, E., Gozzini, B., Marchisio, M., Padoan, J.: Analysis of the thermal comfort in cycling athletes. Proc. Eng. 34, 433–438 (2012)
6. Pezzoli, A., Cristofori, E.: Analisi, previsioni e misure meteorologiche applicate agli sport equestri. In: 10th Congress "New Findings In Equine Practices", pp. 38–43. Centro Internazionale del Cavallo, Italy (2008)
7. Pope, C.A., Dockery, D.W., Spengler, J.D., Raizenne, M.E.: Respiratory health and PM10 pollution. Am. Rev. Respir. Dis. 144(3), 668–674 (1991)
8. Schwartz, J.: Air pollution and hospital admissions for respiratory disease. Epidemiology 7, 20–28 (1996)
9. Pezzoli, A., Cristofori, E., Moncalero, M., Giacometto, F., Boscolo, A.: Effect of the environment on the sport performance. In: Proceeding of International Congress on Sports Science Research and Technology Support, pp. 167–170. SCITEPRESS, Lisbon (2013)
10. Lobozewicz, T.: Meteorology in Sport. Sportverlag, Frankfurt (1981)
11. Kay, J., Vamplew, W.: Weather Beaten: Sport in the British Climate. Mainstream Publishing, London (2002)
12. Haddon, W.: Options for the prevention of motor vehicle crash injury. Isr. Med. J. 16, 45–65 (1980)

13. Pezzoli, A., Vercelli, G., Boscolo, A., Dalla Vedova, D., Besi, M.: La connessione mente-corpo-ambiente e materiali: una strada nella ricerca della performance? In: XIX Congresso Nazionale AIPS – Il Comportamento Motorio e Sportivo tra Ricerca e Lavoro sul Campo, p. 54. Università degli Studi di Verona – Facoltà di Scienze Motorie, Verona (2012)
14. Arpino, M., Pezzoli, A.: La connsessione mente-corpo-ambiente e materiali nello sport: una strada nella ricerca della performance? SdS 95, 3–14 (2012)
15. Bellasio, R., Maffeis, G., Scire, J., Longoni, M.G., Bianconi, R., Quaranta, N.: Algorithms to account for topographic shading effects and surface temperature dependence on terrain elevation in diagnostic meteorological models. Bound.-Layer Meteorol. 11, 595–614 (2005)
16. OpenStreetMap. http://www.openstreetmap.org
17. Leung, Y.K., Yip, K.M., Yeung, K.H.: Relationship between thermal index and mortality in Hong Kong. Meteorol. Appl. 15, 399–409 (2008)
18. Robaa, S.M.: Effect of urbanization and industrialization processes on outdoor thermal human comfort in Egypt. Atmos. Clim. Sci. 1, 100–112 (2011)
19. Wagner, W.: Surface tension. How temperature sensors can help Olympic ski racers. Meteorol. Tech. Int. 90–93 (2010)
20. Opatkiewicz, A., Williams, T., Walters, C.: The effects of temperature, travel and time off on Major League soccer team performance. In: World Congress of Performance Analysis of Sport IX, Worcester, UK (2012)
21. Brocherie, F., Girard, O., Millet, G.P.: The influence of environmental temperature on home advantage in Qatari International soccer matches. In: World Congress of Performance Analysis of Sport IX, Worcester, UK (2012)
22. Brocherie, F., Girard, O., Farooq, A., Millet, G.P.: Climatic influence on home advantage in Gulf Region Football. Statistical analysis using international match outcomes. In: Proceedings of International Congress on Sports Science Research and Technology Support. SCITEPRESS, Lisbon (2013)
23. Pepino, A.: Abbigliamento e comfort termico nella performance sportiva. MSc thesis in sport science, S.U.I.S.M. – Università di Torino (2012)
24. Moncalero, M., Colonna, M., Pezzoli, A., Nicotra, M.: Pilot study for the evaluation of the thermal properties and moisture management on ski boots. In: Proceedings of International Congress on Sports Science Research and Technology Support, pp. 171–179. SCITEPRESS, Lisbon (2013)

Video-Based Soccer Ball Detection
in Difficult Situations

Josef Halbinger and Juergen Metzler[✉]

Fraunhofer Institute of Optronics, System Technologies and Image Exploitation
IOSB, Fraunhoferstr. 1, 76131 Karlsruhe, Germany
juergen.metzler@iosb.fraunhofer.de
http://www.iosb.fraunhofer.de

Abstract. The interest in video-based systems for acquiring and analyzing player and ball data of soccer games is increasing in several domains such as media and professional training. Consequently, tracking systems for live acquisition of quantitative motion data are becoming widely used. The interest for such systems is especially high for training purposes but the demands concerning the precision of the data are very high. Current systems reach a satisfying precision due to heavy interaction of operators. In order to increase the level of automation while retaining a constantly high precision, more robust tracking systems are required. However, this demand is accompanied by an increasing trend to stand-alone, mobile, low-cost soccer tracking systems due to cost concerns, stadium infrastructure, media rights etc. As a consequence, the live data acquisition has to be accomplished by using only a few cameras so that there are generally only few perspectives of the players and the ball. In addition, only low-resolution images are available in many cases. The low-resolution images strongly exacerbate the problem of detection and tracking the soccer ball. Apart from the challenge that arises from the appearance of the ball, situations where the ball is occluded by the players make the detection of the ball difficult. The lower the number of the cameras is, the lower generally is the number of available perspectives - and thus the more difficult it is to gather precise motion data. This paper presents a soccer ball detection approach that is applicable to difficult situations such as occluded cases. It handles low-resolution images from single static camera systems and can be used e.g. for ball trajectory reconstruction. The performance of the approach is analyzed on a data set of a Bundesliga match.

Keywords: Soccer · Sport analysis · Ball detection · Video-tracking system

1 Introduction

The increasing professionalization of soccer is accompanied by a growing media attention as well as game analysis and professional training. Especially, the automation of live analysis of soccer games is interesting for several domains such as media. This, however, requires a robust acquisition of player and ball

© Springer International Publishing Switzerland 2015
J. Cabri et al. (Eds.): icSPORTS 2013, CCIS 464, pp. 17–24, 2015.
DOI: 10.1007/978-3-319-17548-5_2

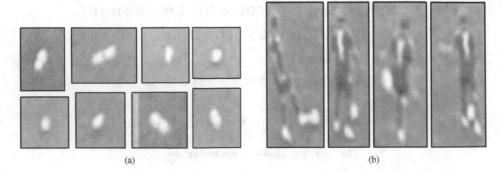

Fig. 1. (a) Variety of the appearance of the ball extracted from one image sequence and (b) examples for partially occluded situations.

data that still relies heavily on the interaction of operators (so-called scouts) in current systems. Live acquisition of quantitative motion data such as distances covered by players, distances between players or ball possession can only be done by sophisticated automation. Our overall two-camera tracking system (one camera per half of the pitch) provides this kind of quantitative data for supporting a scout and for the automated acquisition of the relevant data [1]. It automatically detects, classifies and tracks the ball, the 22 soccer players, the referee and the two linesmen in one stitched image sequence of approximately double Full HD resolution.

The main contribution of this work is the detection of the ball in situations in which the ball is close to a player or even partially covered by one. Detection of the ball in image sequences generally is a difficult task as the appearance of the ball varies from image to image. For instance, the high accelerations occurring at the ball may cause motion blur so that the shape of the ball is then more of an ellipse than a circle (see Fig. 1(a)). In addition, the color of the ball may vary from image to image due to changes of the illumination conditions. It might also have the same color as the lines of the pitch which exacerbates the ball detection task. Another challenge is the image resolution of the ball which is usually very small so that confusions with player body parts may occur. Depending on the camera perspective, the ball is in front of a complex image background such as the audience which exacerbates its detection as well. Besides difficulties that arise from the appearance of the ball itself, the detection of the ball is very challenging in situations where it is occluded by the players (see Fig. 1(b)). Every time a player touches the ball there is a chance that the ball is not fully visible for a short time as parts of the player's body can move between ball and the camera. However, as long as the ball is at least partially visible, there is an opportunity to identify the ball in the image.

The motivation of this work is to find a solution which can help to detect the ball in such cases. At the first stage, a circle detection method is applied. At the second stage, the detected circles are evaluated by examining the Freeman chain code [6] of the found contours. There are several publications for detecting and tracking the soccer ball as seen in [2]. However, most of these approaches focus on

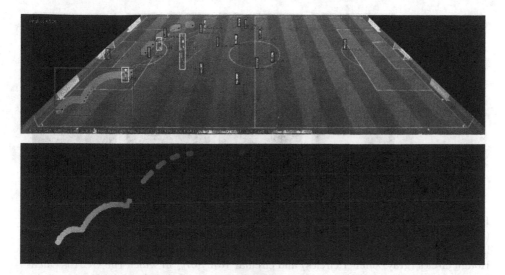

Fig. 2. Sample snapshot of the processed input image sequence including detected ball tracklets marked by rectangles (top) and one for the corresponding motion history image (bottom).

tracking the ball in broadcast soccer videos and require a high image resolution [3]. The approach presented in this contribution is applicable to static camera systems, even for low-resolution cameras. So it can be used in huge tracking systems consisting of several cameras usually fixed installed in stadiums as well as for low-cost tracking systems that generally consist of 1–3 cameras capturing the entire pitch.

The contribution is structured as follows: In Sect. 2, the module for the ball detection is described. It is a two-stage approach: At the first stage, the ball is detected in situations in which it is generally not occluded. Robust partial ball trajectories (tracklets) are extracted. In order to acquire detection hypotheses in occluded situations (within the gaps between the tracklets), a ball detector specialized for occluded situations is used at the second stage. Then, in Sect. 3, results of an evaluation on data sets of a Bundesliga match are presented.

2   Ball Detection

The reconstruction of the ball trajectory requires a reliable soccer ball detection. However, this is challenging as there are usually a lot of occlusions. Furthermore, a high detection rate should be achieved at a low false alarm rate. We follow a detection approach that has been widely established in order to be able to fulfill this requirement (see e.g. [2]): the detection task is divided into two stages in which ball candidates are extracted and verified. First stage: in not occluded situations the ball is detected and confirmed by its appearance as a single object. Second stage: if there is a (partially) occluded situation which means that the ball has not been detected as a single object, a two-step approach is applied that first detects circles in the image and then analyzes the Freeman chain code [6].

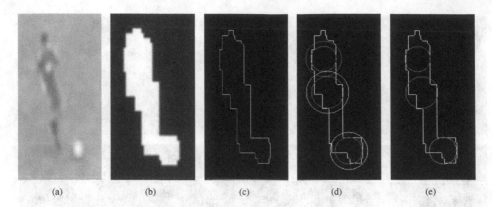

(a)   (b)   (c)   (d)   (e)

Fig. 3. (a) Input image, (b) foreground/background segmentation of the input image, (c) chain code representation of the outer contour: *left-* and *right*-values (yellow and light blue/horizontal lines) of the chain code are of particular interest, (d) detected Hough circles (gray/smaller circles) and circular RoI RoI_{bc} in which the CCH is calculated (blue/upper, brown/central and yellow/lower circle), (e) detected Hough circles and identified ball (green/lower cirlce) (Color figure online).

2.1 Not Occluded Situations

At the first stage, the soccer ball has to be detected as a single object. Due to the real-time constraint for live applications, a feature-based detection with e.g. a sliding windows approach cannot be used. Instead, as the images from a static camera are captured, the foreground/background segmentation from Kim et al. [4] is applied at first. Temporal static background like the pitch and marking lines are segmented as background, whereas moving objects generate changing appearance and are therefore segmented as foreground. During the ball candidate extraction, all foreground regions are extracted and checked for their size using calibration information of the cameras. Foreground regions that are no candidates for the soccer ball due to their size are removed. Out of the remaining regions, the external contours are extracted as a sequence of points and analyzed afterwards. If the number of the contour pixels is higher than a specific bias, an ellipse is fitted to it and the mean squared error between every sequence point and the ellipse is calculated. Ball candidates with a high mean squared error are removed. The remaining candidates are kept as verified foreground regions in the foreground/background segmented image. Then, a dilatation is applied and the last n binary images are accumulated to a so-called Motion History Image (MHI) of verified ball candidates. Finally, ball tracklets (robust partial ball trajectories) are finally extracted from the MHI. Figure 2 shows a MHI and some results of detected/extracted ball tracklets.

2.2 Partially Occluded Situations

The foreground/background segmentation of the first stage often merges ball and player into a single silhouette if they are either close to each other or partially occlude each other. Thus, the ball is not a singular object and only appears as a bump poking out of the player's silhouette in the resulting image (Fig. 3(a) and (b)).

At the second stage, the goal is to identify these bumps. In order to achieve this, we apply a two-step approach again. In the first step, circles (or at least parts of circles) in the image are detected via Hough transform [5]. In the second step, the Freeman chain code is considered to decide if a detected circle is a soccer ball.

In the following, the details of the procedure are given: At the beginning of the first step, all the player silhouettes of the foreground/background segmented image are extracted into separate images. On each of these silhouette images, a Hough transform for circle detection is applied. All detected circles and circular arcs that approximately match the predefined ball dimensions are determined as ball candidates. A resulting Hough circle c is characterized by the center coordinates x and y as well as the radius $r : c = (x, y, r)$.

The Hough transform variant chosen in this work is called the Hough gradient method [7]. Unlike comparable methods, this variant only uses a two-dimensional accumulator instead of a three dimensional one. This is achieved by incrementing only accumulator cells along the gradient direction of each non zero pixel of the edge map instead of incrementing a complete circle and therefore keeping a separate accumulator for every predefined possible circle radius. This is beneficial to the running time of the algorithm. The downside is a lower recognition rate of circles with a concentric counterpart. But this flaw is acceptable since concentric circles do not occur in the segmented image material.

At the beginning of the second step, the outer contour of the silhouette image is calculated. Then the Freeman chain code of the contour is determined (Fig. 3(c)). Now, in a circular Region of Interest (RoI) around the ball candidates that were identified before, the Chain Code Histogram (CCH) is computed [8].

The circular RoI is constructed around the center coordinates x and y of the ball candidate, adding a small Δ to the radius r (Fig. 3(d)). The Δ is added to encounter the problem that the detected circles of the Hough gradient method tend to be slightly smaller than they actually are. As a result, the considered RoI around the ball candidate RoI_{bc} is defined as $RoI_{bc} = (x, y, r + \Delta)$.

As described in [8], the CCH is a discrete function

$$p(k) = \frac{n_k}{n}, k = 0, 1, ..., K - 1, \tag{1}$$

where n_k is the number of chain code values k in a chain code, and n is the number of links in a chain code. In case of the Freeman chain code there are $K = 8$ possible directions.

Generally, a bump has a high amount of $left$ and $right$-values of the chain code at the same time, while the $left$-values are on the upper side of the bump and $right$-values on the lower side of the bump. As a consequence, a RoI_{bc} with a CCH that provides certain frequencies of occurrence of $left$- and $right$-values λ and ρ is defined to indicate a bump in the silhouette. If this frequency lies beyond a certain threshold τ (and RoI_{bc} originates from inside the silhouette), it is assumed that a bump exists in this area. As this bump also matches the dimensions of the soccer ball, the examined RoI_{bc} is identified to have the soccer ball in it (Fig. 3(e)):

$$Ball = \begin{cases} 1 & : \lambda \geq \tau \quad \text{and} \quad \rho \geq \tau \\ 0 & : else \end{cases}. \tag{2}$$

3   Experimental Results

We tested the first-stage of our approach - the tracklet extraction - on a data set of a Bundesliga match consisting of an image sequence with about 140.000 images of double Full HD resolution (see Fig. 2 for an example). There are 1428 tracklets to detect, in situations where the ball is neither occluded nor merged with a player. In these situations the approach detected 1343 tracklets and missed 85. There was no false alarm, i.e. all detected ball tracklets were correctly detected as such.

The second-stage - ball detection in occluded situations - was tested on two data sets of a Bundesliga match. Both sets consist of image regions that were extracted from the same Bundesliga sequence as in the first stage test. The first data set consists of 1408 non-consecutive images with a resolution of 50×100 pixels, 704 of them showing the ball close to a player or partially occluded by

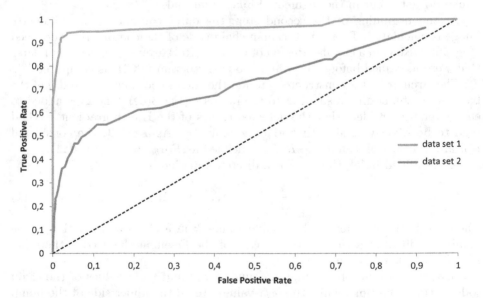

Fig. 4. ROC curve of the tested second-stage approach: the ball detection approach for occluded situations. "data set 1" consists of 1408 non-consecutive images: 704 of them showing the ball close to a player or partially occluded by a player and the other 704 images don't show a ball. "data set 2" consists of 9634 consecutive images: 111 of them showing the ball close to a player or partially occluded by a player and 9323 images don't show the ball.

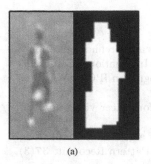 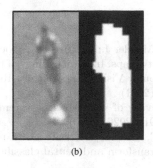 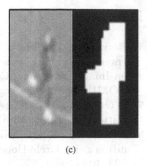

(a)   (b)   (c)

Fig. 5. Difficult cases for the ball detector: (a) Ball between player's legs, (b) ball right in front of a player and (c) player without a ball, although there is a bump in the segmented image.

a player. The other 704 images don't show a ball. The second data set consists of 9634 consecutive images with a resolution of 64×128 pixels, 111 of them showing the ball close to a player or partially occluded by a player. 9323 images don't show the ball.

As mentioned in Sect. 2.2, the threshold τ describes the required frequencies of occurrence λ and ρ of $left$ and $right$ chain code values inside of RoI_{bc}. In order to determine the optimal threshold, τ is iterated from a specified minimum to a specified maximum in both data sets. The range is set in a way that all possible cases are covered: it starts with a configuration that identifies every Hough circle as a ball and ends with a configuration that detects no single Hough circle as a ball. The results are displayed in a ROC (Receiver Operating Characteristics) curve that puts the true positive rate of a data set in relationship with its false positive rate (see Fig. 4).

In the second data set, a true positive respectively false positive rate of 1.0 could not be reached. The reason for this is that no Hough circles matching the predefined ball dimensions were found. This leads to scenarios where varying the τ-threshold has no effect. The results also differ because the second data set has more difficult cases: On the one hand, there are several images in which the ball is between the player's legs as illustrated in Fig. 5(a) or right in front of the foot as shown in Fig. 5(b). As a result, the ball does not appear as a bump in the segmented image. On the other hand, there are segmented images that have a strong bump, although there is no ball on the input image as shown in Fig. 5(c).

4 Conclusions

In this paper, a two-stage approach for the detection of the soccer ball has been presented. The focus is on occluded situations in which the ball is partially occluded or merged with a player. We could yield a reliable extraction of ball tracklets in not occluded situations. Also, the ball detector for occluded situations is able to reliably detect balls in cases where the ball is partially occluded. With the exception of the delay in the output of the ball coordinates, which depends on the length of the motion history, the proposed approach is real-time capable.

References

1. Herrmann, C., Manger, D., Metzler J.: Feature-based localization refinement of players in soccer using plausibility maps. In: Proceedings of the International Conference on Image Processing, Computer Vision, and Pattern Recognition IPCV (WORLD-COMP), vol. 2, Las Vegas (2011)
2. D'Orazi, T., Leo, M.: A review of vision-based systems for soccer video analysis. Pattern Recognit. **43**(8), 2911–2926 (2010)
3. D'Orazi, T., Guaragnella, C., Leo, M., Distante, A.: A new algorithm for ball recognition using circle Hough transform and neural classifier. Pattern Recognit. **37**(3), 393–408 (2004)
4. Kim, K., Chalidabhongse, T.H., Harwood, D., Davis, L.: Real-time foreground-background segmentation using codebook model. Real-Time Imag. Spec. Iss. Video Object Process. **11**(3), 172–185 (2004)
5. Kimme, C., Ballard, D., Sklansky, J.: Finding circles by an array of accumulators. Commun. ACM **18**(2), 120–122 (1975)
6. Freeman, H.: On the encoding of arbitrary geometric configurations. IRE Trans. Electron. Comput. EC **10**(2), 260–268 (1961)
7. Bradski, G., Kaehler, A.: Learning OpenCV: Computer Vision with the OpenCV Library. O'Reilly Media, Sebastopol (2008)
8. Iivarinen, J., Visa, A.J.E.: Shape recognition of irregular objects. Proc. SPIE **2904**, 25–32 (1996)

Application and UI Design for Ergonomic Heart Rate Monitoring in Endurance Sports: Realizing an Improved Tool for Health and Sports Activities on Base of Android Smartphone Programming and ANT+

Hans Weghorn[(⊠)]

BW Cooperative State University, Kronenstrasse 53A, 70174 Stuttgart, Germany
weghorn@dhbw-stuttgart.de

Abstract. During endurance sports training, heart rate conveniently can be used as proportional measure for the current physical effort of an on-going workout. Accordingly, it is advantageous during such exercises to obtain monitoring information about the actual heart rate for having an instrument of controlling the demand level of an activity. Today, the market offers a broad variety of sports computers, which allow display and tracking of heart rate, but their usability and appropriateness appear rather limited in terms of an efficient application in daily training. In particular, major restrictions are numerical displays of the in-time measures with tiny letters or an unfiltered print-out of spurious values, since the recording is not always precise, but sometimes disturbed from various reasons. Fortunately, upcoming new technologies like programmable smartphone devices and ANT+ communication standard for sports sensors do allow developing new and optimized applications and systems also for sports and health purposes. In the work here, a convenient heart rate monitor was developed that aims at improved user-friendliness in combination with elaborated signal-conditioning for preventing any spurious and misguiding displays. Few simple button presses put the sportsman into the position of performing efficiently activities within the desired endurance training range. As result, a system is described that is feasible for easy-to-use and efficient sports monitoring, especially during daily workouts.

Keywords: Heart rate monitor · Endurance training · UI · Android · ANT+

1   Introduction

For physical sports and health activities it is important to know the actual blood oxygen supply level for categorizing such activities into the effects of regeneration, aerobic and anaerobic training. This is required, because then only dedicate training units will lead in a controlled and predictable manner to the desired training goals [1], for instance building up speed, over-all endurance or muscular strength. In practical sports medicine, blood is extracted from the training person and the analysis of its lactate concentration yields the state of the oxygen supply, but this method obviously is too complicate and too expensive for being continuously applied as monitoring instrument in daily training units.

© Springer International Publishing Switzerland 2015
J. Cabri et al. (Eds.): icSPORTS 2013, CCIS 464, pp. 25–41, 2015.
DOI: 10.1007/978-3-319-17548-5_3

Fortunately, an alternative measure, which is applicable at much better convenience, has been identified since long time: monitoring of the heart rate (HR) allows a replacement of the direct measure of the blood oxygen level by a proportional value [2]. More precisely, as established measure the percentage value of the actual heart rate in relation to the maximal possible heart rate (HR_{max}) of the individual sports person is used. Consequently, this kind of monitoring approach is commonly applied for field investigations in medical science [3] and also in sports research [4]. Figure 1 provides a sketch of the main sports activity levels as these are mapped to different bands of heart rate.

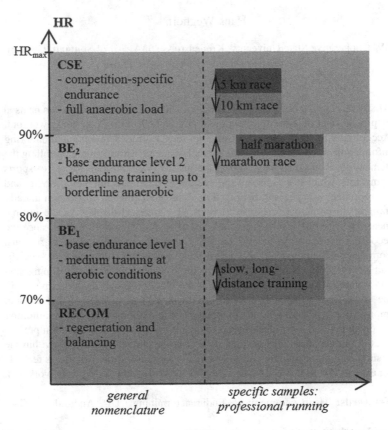

Fig. 1. Activity categories as function of HR_{max} (the maximal individual heart rate).

For beginners in sports – especially, older ones – it is established practice that they first build up their base performance in range RECOM and then after sufficient advance continue within BE_1, since exceeding these levels could even be hazardous for such untrained people. In general, efficient sport training requires a certain, well-known mixture of these activities levels in Fig. 1. Else there won't be any power advance or even physical deterioration may arise after reaching a certain endurance level despite continued high training efforts.

As sample reference, Fig. 1 exposes also some typical ranges for different running activities in the right column, while the left column in the table applies to human sports activities in general.

Electronic consumer market offers today a big variety of devices for HR monitoring (Fig. 2). This ranges from rather simple and cheap watches to elaborated sports computers. All of them are tiny, wearable devices, but their ergonomy in terms of user interfacing (UI) appears rather low, when considering fundamental knowledge and experience for the research field of human computer interaction (HCI). For instance, usually the actual heart rate count is printed in letters of limited size and often with limited contrast on B+W displays. This invokes two fundamental problems, since this kind of output is

- readable at a low speed only
- must be categorized by the training persons themselves (refer to Fig. 1)

Certainly, people usually claim that they can easily remember the desired limits for their workout in terms of lower and upper heart rate count. In training practice, after longer time of demanding activities, the true experience is quite different: even the comparison of the simple numbers will get really slow and causes considerable extra efforts, after, for instance, attending several hours in a distance run.

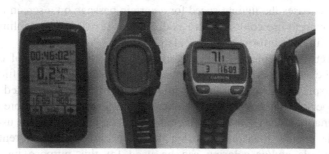

Fig. 2. Typical sports computers and watches, which can perform heart rate monitoring as main feature or in addition to other functionalities.

Another effect is, that the measuring results from the heart sensor are sometimes disturbed for spurious reasons, and displayed totally unfiltered by the sports watches. In general, systematic errors in the sensor information have been reported recently for such sports devices [5].

The actual trend of the HR – in particular the question, whether the heart is getting slowly too high or too low – is particularly relevant for efficiently controlling an on-going workout. Despite this interrelation, the HR trend has to be traced manually by the sports user, while observing HR number display of the sports computer and calculating then the slope "by hand".

There are also already modern UI concepts implemented in some commercial devices. For instance, certain sports computers allow to program limits for a monitoring of the lower and upper HR during the workouts, and there is even a haptic warning signal generated, since these devices start vibrating, if one of these limits is exceeded.

In daily use, it unfortunately turns out that exactly this feature is worthless, because the unfiltered HR measures spuriously produce such warning signals. Furthermore, the warning signal in the sports watch is often identically for the events of too low and too high values. This makes it impossible to interpret the haptic notification correctly. Further reading of a message is required that is then displayed in even smaller letters, since the corresponding printout carries more information and requires more characters that have to map on the tiny screen.

From fundamental HCI research it can be derived, that information perception in computerized displays can be accelerated by different principles:

- Using color as information indicator [6]
- Using analogue graphics instead of values that are in printed in letters

As standard knowledge from the use of technical systems it is suggested that analogue tachometers are read approx. three times faster than digitally displayed ones. Although investigations from the modern application field of automotive do not proof this number as precise value [7], they do support the general theory that analogue displays are perceived at least as fast, by tendency even faster than digital ones.

As complementing UI aspect, the benefit of coloring texts is well know and has been investigated thoroughly during the time, when colored computer displays became affordable and were widely commercialized. Systematic research has shown that the use of colors increases the finding speed for a certain passage on a screen [8]. The best scheme was found to use colors that are as distinct as possible for enabling the fastest perception of different information contents [9].

For the user's convenience, the categorization and the detection of out-of-band-trends could be easily performed by the sports computers and data filtering could prevent the display of erroneous or misguiding outputs. The calculated results and trends, and especially the commands, whether the training should be more challenging or slower for mapping the desired working range, can be indicated to the user in a more easily readable manner than just exposing the plain digits of the current heart rate. Graphical symbols and/or coloring can be used for this purpose instead of text printouts.

In the following sections, the considerations and deductions are discussed that guided to the design and construction of an appropriate heart rate monitor that is intended for sports and health exercises. First scope was an improved UI that meets standards according to the established knowledge from the field of HCI. Second focus was a general improvement of signal processing, which is described in the next section, as it depicts the base for the whole UI concept.

A relevant part of the improvement is also that the person, who uses this device, is not required to know all the numbers and relations of sports training categories, but simple button presses inside the application allow defining the proper and desired demand level of the workout. Accordingly, the system is even more valuable for beginners and in sports endurance trainings.

2 Signal Conditioning of Heart Rate Data

2.1 Low-Pass Filtering of Input Stream

For the detection of heart activities, the use of special chest straps has been established and commercialized. Such products work really reliable also for long time of continuous use. Commonly, the signals are recorded from two skin electrodes across the lower chest, and are then processed by a tiny hardware module on the belt that transmits the result via RF to any data processing sink.

In the experiments here, a comfort chest strap of the manufacturer Garmin Ltd. was used, its RF transmission is composed in accordance to the ANT+ standard [10] that is discussed in the following section about technical aspects.

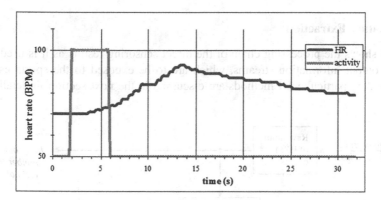

Fig. 3. Experiment on the slope of the heart rate. After slight warming up, three pull-ups are completed while holding breath during the plotted activity window (rectangular curve). The heart rate responds by a gradual increase with delay, while the relaxation phase follows at an even slower remission speed.

The used sensor produces four raw measures per second, a sampling rate that is typical for such chest straps. The observation is that sometime these HR measures appear spuriously distorted, the reasons have not scientifically been investigated yet, but are suspected being manifold, e.g., the electrode contacts are not always accurate due to body movements, electronic problems, and RF disturbances.

The dedicate reasons may vary, of importance is mainly, how further processing can overcome such effects of falsified input data. A standard solution in signal processing is averaging consecutive measures as this stands for filtering the effect of such unavoidable and unpredictable short-term disturbances. The properties of such a low-pass filter have to be aligned to the physiological behavior of the human body in general, since averaging in terms of any low-pass filtering will suppress the slope of the output signal and may therefore lead to wrong macroscopic measures, which would automatically consequence wrong instructions for any on-going training activities.

Medical research is much older than mobile computer technology, and hence, base investigations about the slope of the HR under certain influencing conditions can be found already from the last century [11]. In this extreme, but indicative experiment, stopping breath followed by physical effort showed already that the body reaction in terms of increasing heart beat rate after sudden load events may be delayed in the order of seconds.

This easily can also be verified with modern computer technology like in the practical experiment in Fig. 3 (an engineering version of the HR monitor was used in this test). From both sources, it can be deducted that averaging HR samples within a range of few seconds will still yield sufficient results with adequate slope. Hence, a time slot of 2.5 s, which stands for an averaging frame of ten incoming sensor measures, is applied in the software construction here. A sliding time-window is used, so the averaging stage yields also an output rate of four values per second, which is synchronized to the input data stream.

2.2   Feature Extraction

Figure 4 shows the processing chain of the direct sensoring results as it is used as tier for four output information streams, which are to be exposed to the sports user (the corresponding particular UI methods are discussed in the next section in detail).

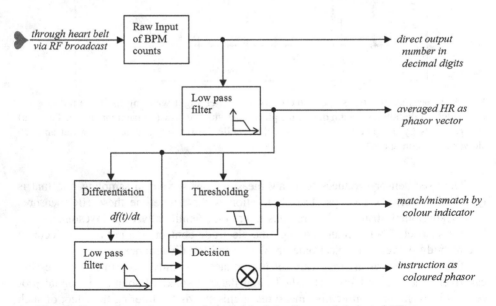

Fig. 4. Generation and consumption model of the direct and deducted HR measures.

In accordance to the different output indicators, the HR has to be compared to thresholds. For instance, if a 60 years old person wants to perform exercises at the effort level of BE_1, the heart rate should typically remain within the band from 119 to 136 beats per second. This mapping yields one important control information.

Of further relevance is the current trend in an on-going activity, more precisely the observation, whether there is a trend that the exercises are running out of the desired band. Such an evolvement can be detected by differentiating the averaged HR curve. The derived slope indicates, whether the pulse is getting too low or too high.

In workout practice, there will often be a slope that is non-zero, but the relevant matter is, whether the value is going to truly run out of band. With human as part of a control loop, correction indicators have to be applied carefully; else over-reaction easily may produce an undesired oscillation in the system. In general it is difficult to set a precise level of physical effort, although the body control can improve with growing experience.

Hence, for out-of-band trends it makes sense to have two stages of indication: first level is just exposing the current situation (applied when there is only slight decrease or increase) without any further instruction. The second is to more clearly indicate the wrong evolvement and combine it with a particular instruction for the activity like asking to slow down or speed up.

For the technically and medically interested user the unfiltered heart rate measure may also be of relevance, and accordingly the value is printed as digital number on the screen. This corresponds additionally to the fact that the heart rate value is the main information, which is commonly exposed in commercial HR monitors or HR apps for sports tracking. In summary, this analysis of data processing yields four output information streams for a display to the user: the raw data sequence and three filtered and processed derivatives of it.

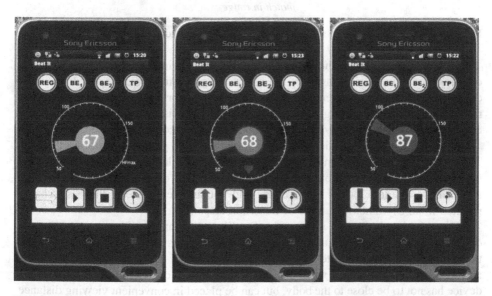

Fig. 5. Collection of photographs of output screens for different use situations. As seen here, the UI is constructed in a self-explaining way. For testing of the output color scheme, the MHR was set to a non-physiological value of 100 bpm for the right two test images (Colour figure online).

3   Optimization of the User Interface

3.1   Visualization of Outputs

The primary goal of the user interface is to provide an information display that is as clear and as quick and effortless readable as possible. This display shall expose the situation and provide instructions of how to behave for staying within or – in case there is a mismatch already – for getting back to the desired training stress level.

As known from many other applications like, e.g., car driving and weather stations, an analogue tachometer is used as main display for the actual heart rate (Fig. 5). The phase vector inside the tachometer circle is controlled by the averaged HR, the corresponding indexing hand is drawn intentionally big for achieving high and quick readability. The indexing hand is painted in color.

By that, the information, which is to be controlled most often for an efficient workout, is visualized: bright green exposes that the heart rate is within the desired stress level band. If the HR drops too much, this color turns to blue, if it is getting too high, it turns to red. In this color indicator, the rule of readability was infringed intentionally: there are not only the three, very distinct colors of green, blue, and red in the scheme, but the transition between these color states is smoothed.

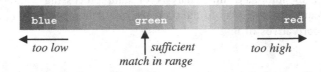

Fig. 6. Color transition scheme for indicating the match or a gradual mismatch of the heart rate.

Like explained before, the human is a critical factor in the control loop, because over-reaction could arise easily by wrong reading or interpretation of displays: it doesn't make sense to suddenly turn the display indicator for the non-mapping heart rate from bright green to bright red, if the range is just missed by one single or a few counts, because this certainly would provoke too strong corrections.

As result, the slope of this indicator is smoothed by a gradual transition of colors. This scheme was experimented manually with the display appearance of the used smartphone, since it turned out that a straight calculation of ramping up and down of the RGB base colors looked inconvenient and not sufficiently sleek; the best scheme resulted in an asymmetric number of transition steps (Fig. 6).

The raw data value, as it is received unfiltered from the chest strap sensor, is displayed in big letters and at high contrast. If the sports user really wants to know this information from time to time, it is thus read easily also from a distance. This appears useful, for instance, when any type of ergometer or treadmill is used, and the device has not to be close to the body, but can be placed in convenient viewing distance and direction. In such cases it even can be avoided to turn the head from the normal workout position for perceiving the information like it is required with built-in displays of such sports apparatuses, which are often mounted ponderable below chest height.

Table 1. Use hierarchy of display information.

Indicator for	UI mode	Frequency of use	Perception time
HR inside range	Color/analogue	~1 /min	≪1 s
HR value	Phasor/analogue	>1 /min	~1 s
Instruction	Colored phasor	>1 /min	~1 s
Precise HR	Number print	Rare	>1 s

Just for technical information, a blinking heart symbol indicates that the RF link to the heart beat sensor is working correctly (located in Fig. 5 below the tachometer centre). If the system detects that the HR is going to exceed the defined limits, another UI element is activated as indicator. A pointer is tilted upwards or downwards, which stands for the instruction to speed up or slow down with the on-going effort respectively (effect is visible in the right two photographs in Fig. 5). Depending on the strength of the wrong trend, the phasor is tinted more or less in red tones.

Table 1 summarizes the reading hierarchy, which stands in accordance to the use frequency of the information puzzle pieces for dedicatedly controlling a workout.

3.2 Efficient Input Controls

Totally new in this construction is a convenient selection of input controls and it is thus the third big improvement in comparison to commercial heart rate monitors (Fig. 2). As listed in Fig. 7, a set of quick buttons is available on top UI screen, through which the user can set the monitoring level according to Fig. 1. For this, it is required that the HR_{max} is configured once in the application (accessible through standard settings menu like is implemented in all smartphone apps).

As control base the HR_{max} parameter appears critical. Best would be, if it is determined under supervision of an experienced doctor. There are many, different formulas in various sports discussions panels found on the Internet as also in various research papers. The two described main methods, which yield slightly different results, are based on the age of the person. No valid scientific foundation for these calculation rules was found in literature, and hence the sports user is not offered in the heart monitor here to enter the age, since the automatic calculation of a wrong HR_{max} could be risky or at least lead to inefficient training ranges.

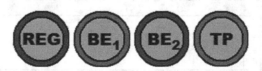

Fig. 7. Quick buttons design for setting the desired training effort level – collection of active and in-active screen buttons. Their activation is indicated by a brightly shining green ring (refer to use cases in Fig. 5) (Color figure online).

The quick buttons for the effort level simplify the control considerably. According to the invoked function behind, it is not required, that a sports user does know all the relations between training goals and heart rates, and the system also releases the sports user from continuously validating in his head, whether the HR maps like desired. Besides the standard effort levels, there is also a button for activating a dedicate training plan. This initiates a well-defined sequence of varying effort levels; for instance, it may be programmed that the sports user first works 10 min in RECOM, then 10 min in BE_1, then 10 min in BE_2 and before terminating the workout, again 5 min in BE_1. Of course, such a plan has to be entered with all its stages into the system, but this method is required for advanced sports training anyway.

There is one button for activating the RF link to the heart belt, which is of technical function. If the air link is active, a beating heart symbol inside the HR tachometer indicates the working connection (Fig. 5). Further buttons are available on screen for training control: the start button initiates a continuous recording of HR samples and it can also be used for pausing, while the stop button allows terminating and closing a workout file (low part of the UI screens in Fig. 5).

At the moment, the recording is stored to a XML-coded file on the multi-media card of the phone. From there, it can be directly downloaded into any compatible sports evaluation software, which is running on a personal computer (e.g. the Garmin training center, or similar others). On the personal computer, the records can then be analyzed and archived for a long-term planning and trace of workout activities. If the GPS signal is available, the heart rate records are also tagged with GPS position information (result of a biking test lap visible in Fig. 8). Since the XML format is not space saving, the

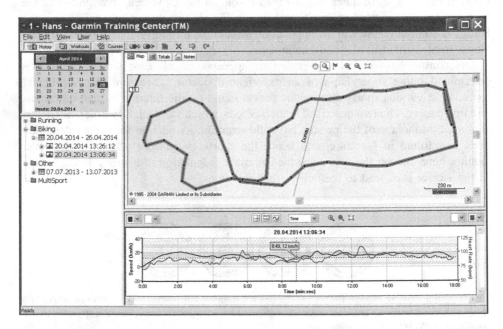

Fig. 8. Recording the GPS trace is implemented in the HR monitor as side feature. For limiting the size of the workout files, track points are recorded coarsely, but the elapsed distance is accumulated with full precision of the GPS module. As seen here, such workouts can be easily imported into a personal sports data base like, e.g., the product of the company Garmin Ltd.

GPS tagging is performed at a reduced rate (four samples per minute) to keep the total files size within reasonable limits, but the total distance is traced and accumulated with highest sampling resolution of the GPS module.

All the control buttons are designed as "self-expressive", which is achieved by using standard nomenclature and commonly used standard symbols.

4 Summary Discussion on Working State

4.1 Base Concept and Application Scenarios

From well-known fundamentals of HCI research, the described approach of constructing a user-friendly heart rate monitor arises partially as straight-forward design. Of course, certain detail questions (e.g. transition scheme for color indicators, averaging duration of raw data input) had to be researched in literature and complemented by dedicate practical experiments.

Since this HR monitor represents a versatile tool and is not specific to any particular kind of sports, it can be used broadly. Especially, endurance exercises and training – and by that building up general physical fitness in sports or health – is the best field for its application. The smartphone can be mounted on a bicycle or on any type of sports machine in a way that it is easily visible by the user without unnatural movements of the head. Although training utilities like, e.g., treadmills and cycloergometers usually have built-in heart rate monitoring as well, these devices do often not work easily or even do not work at all with custom heart chest straps. At least, there is a procedure for registering a personal strap and – furthermore, if a personal one cannot be used – there may remain hygienic concerns when sharing such a skin touching belt with other people. After the workout it is often not possible to get access to the records of the training that is stored inside the computer of the sports apparatus.

Hence, using an own HR monitor on such gymnastic machines provides in total several advantages, namely the opportunity for a natural and comfortable use during the training, hygienic advantages and the possibility for easily preserving the records of the workout for later analysis and planning.

4.2 Technical Realization Aspects

Considering the practical implementation of the HR monitor, the possibilities can be compared to the evolvement of mobile phones in their first generations, since sports watches and computers are nowadays also closed technical systems, regardless whether they are simple or elaborated. Neither their functionality, nor their software can be modified. For smartphones, it is meanwhile well established that other people than just their constructors can bring own software applications on these units or can even extend hardware through standard interfaces. For the experiments in this work a smartphone with the "open" operating system Android was chosen [12], since there is lots of developer support and introductory material available in terms of books and on the Internet in documentation and developers panels.

Industry for sports computers has agreed several years ago on a new RF communication standard, which enables the interoperability of devices from different vendors. In the past before, sport device constructors used their proprietary air link solutions, today the so-called ANT+ standard [10] offers an efficient data transfer from typical sensors like heart straps, foot pods for tread detection, or speed sensors for running and cycling. Like Bluetooth (BT) and WLAN, ANT+ uses the ISM frequency band, but at much lower energy consumption, which makes it possible that a heart chest strap can run several days from the energy of one single lithium battery cell.

Since the corresponding working consortium for ANT+ is interested in spreading the standard, it claims that there is a long list of smartphones, which do supply this communication link as well. In the end, the number of phones with built-in ANT+ interface certainly is growing, but nevertheless, it is not really broadly available, if all the available smartphones products are considered.

At the time, when the investigations in this research were started, there were few and expensive ANT+ phones only. In this project, a Sony Xperia Active was selected as target device, it has got an older version of the Android operating system, but it was constructed especially for outdoor and sports use and it comes with a special pocket for wearing it at the forearm or upper arm during such activities (Fig. 9). There is good software support for developers from the phone manufacturer, but the ANT+ application software technology is complicate anyway, and it is proprietary.

With newer versions of smartphone operating systems, there may be some day a built-in standard software interfacing to ANT+. This concept theoretically will allow transferring applications, like the one in this project, more easily to devices of other brands. In the meantime the solution is to install a plug-in service as software bridge to ANT+ hardware on the particular smart phone as it is available on the Internet market places for modern devices. Unfortunately, this requires some special device handling and is not the preferable method for non-technical sports people. New upcoming alternative communication standards like the so-called Smart BT may also open a broader range of target devices for the HR monitor, which is discussed in the next section about future extensions.

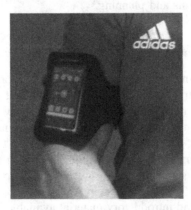

Fig. 9. Upper arm pocket bag as it is part in the delivery package of the outdoor smartphone that was used here. This wearing solution does appear neither comfortable nor useful for any kind of sports activities.

In the context of this work, there is further investigation planned on integrating various sports sensors for generating further versatile control and monitoring tools. This will be continued to a certain extend with the device, which was used here, since the outputs are not intended for any commercial purpose. An update of operating systems and application development versions will be applied as it becomes mandatory, e.g., through the integration of newer device generations like in Fig. 10.

5 Overcoming Concept Constraints by Future Extensions

5.1 Using an Alternative RF Standard

ANT+ represents a well-engineered RF communication standard, which can be used for sports and health devices. Unfortunately, an additional hardware module is required in the terminal unit for serving this link, which is not implemented in each commercial device. On the other hand, modern computer devices do all support BT and a new power-saving version, which is called BT Smart, is currently being introduced especially on the smart phone market. Heart chest straps are also available since longer time with BT Smart as also other sports sensors (Fig. 10). These devices were initially addressing the high-end smart phone segment of one specific vendor.

Meanwhile also Android has a defined support for BT Smart via an improved programming through so-called device profiles [13], the commercial support of this can be widely expected during the next year, while compatible Android versions above level 4 are being introduced on the consumer market. This will enable to evolve the HR monitor, which was developed here, for serving a much increased number of smart phones. The justification for this transfer appears clear when considering the UI screen in Fig. 10, which again documents the inobservance even in very recent market products of all the beneficial UI concepts that were discussed in the sections before.

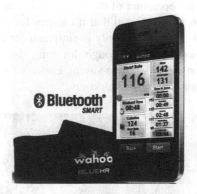

Fig. 10. Smart BT heart chest strap with screen shot of smart phone App for using it.

Conversely, the ANT+ consortium publishes a list for clear advantages over BT smart [14] like, e.g., that the limitation of cell nodes in a BT network certainly will cause considerable interference problems in bigger events, where thousands of sportsmen attend and many of them want to use simultaneously such devices. Without technology preferences and for best convenience, of course, any HR monitor should allow to dynamically allow using both RF links as alternative, so the customers and sports user can decide what to use depending on the particular case and equipment.

5.2 Limitations in Usability

Although the developed HR monitor appears applicable for its intended purpose, it is open to investigate its usability by scientific methods. Obviously, the system has got also some limitations, which arise from its technical construction. For instance – due to the RF communication inside the ISM frequency band – it is unusable for swimming or under/in-water activities.

A smartphone in the end has got some physical dimensions and weight, and hence such a unit will neither be helpful nor appreciated in sports competitions. For this, much smaller and less cramping devices similar to slight watches are required. The same concern arises during daily training in running, cross-country skiing and all other comparable activities, where an extra carrier pouch has to be used (Fig. 9).

Here also very recent mobile technologies like so-called smart watches may help to construct an appropriate solution: watch-like systems can be used as light-weight tool for the sportsmen (Fig. 11). Concerning the system structure, the latter represents a remote display, while the computing power and intelligence is still located inside a smart phone that is worn in a bag close to the body and by that much less disturbing.

In first experiments here, the before described HR monitor was extended by such a remote display, Fig. 11 shows a life image of this system under operation. During practical use it turned out that the wrist display is even more convenient than the sports computers in Fig. 2, because it is lighter and provides better readability because of its color screen and the possibility to program sufficient sizes in digit printouts.

Two critical aspects have been investigated in this design structure, because of their fundamental influence on the operation of the system. First, the operational time of the wrist display was tested and it was found that it can run for approximately three hours under full screen illumination. This certainly is sufficient for average sportsmen, but it has to be stated that it wouldn't be enough for long distance activities like slow marathon or ultra-marathon runs. A power-saving concept for the wrist display would be required to serve also such extreme workouts.

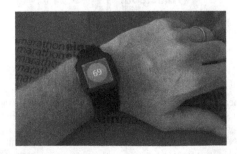

Fig. 11. Remote wrist display for Android smartphone. This device can perfectly complement the heart rate monitoring UI for endurance sports like, e.g., distance running or skating.

The second concern was the RF quality for workout trace, when the smart phone device is carried inside any bags or pockets. Different experiments were conducted on this, in some the smart phone was worn in a side pocket of a sports clothing, in other tests the smartphone was placed even inside a sports rucksack. The tested disciplines were running, skating any bicycling (sample in Fig. 8). In all cases it could be validated with simultaneous use of other sports computers, that the RF link to the HR strap as also the GPS recording was working reliably. E.g., the distance error in the registered workout paths stayed strictly in the order of below 1 % despite it is not a primary feature of the HR monitor to perform GPS tracking at all.

As smart watch technology is also evolving quickly, it can be expected that in future the entire sports tracking software, like the HR monitor here, can be operated on such a single device and no background processing on an additional smart phone will be required. Certainly, a considerable improvement of computing power and battery time is required for these tiny units, so this won't be realizable in near future. Accordingly, the developments here will focus in the next years on the relaying approach for providing even more convenience to sports users of such systems.

5.3 Effect of Cardiodrift in HR Monitoring

Referencing sports physiology, there arises a general question with the concept of linking workouts to the HR_{max}. Especially in endurance training, different energy reservoirs in the human body are used in a sequence. During the first minutes, phosphate storage is used, which is located inside the muscles, and low oxygen is required for burning this. Consequently, the heart rate as indicator for oxygen transport flow is lowered in the beginning of sports activities. After this – for a phase of approx. 1.5 h – the body uses carbohydrate burning, which maps in general well to the HR levels in Fig. 1. Afterwards if the person is used to it, the body tries to supply itself by "fat" burning (i.e. a conversion of fat reservoirs into carbohydrate, which is then used as energy supply for the muscles). In this phase, the heart rate starts increasing considerably, because of a much higher oxygen consumption for this workout stage.

But even in the phase of carbohydrate burning at steady aerobic level, there exists the so-called effect of "cardiodrift" [15]. It stands for a continuous, slight increase of HR, which occurs despite a perfectly balanced demand level already for workouts less than an hour. Cardiodrift is not fully understood yet, there even exists some controversial discussion since longer time about its origin, but the effect itself is not under question and hence, it would to be considered in an accurate training regulation as well. The control loops in the developed HR monitor are not prepared yet for compensating this effect, at the current state of research reports it wouldn't anyway be possible to identify a general mathematical rule for continuously adopting the HR band limits during an on-going workout.

This all implies that HR monitoring doesn't work well as effort indicator for short workouts, and appears only reasonable with a programmed training plan for longer workouts. Without detail knowledge about these relations or planning support and guidance from appropriate experts, HR-controlled training units may have only limited effects, when the workouts are too short or too long.

6 Conclusions and Outlook

The concept of a user-friendly heart rate monitor has been researched scientifically, and it has been realized on base of the corresponding findings technically. In this system, colored and analogue display indicators allow perceiving the most relevant heart monitoring information with quick and effortless glances in less than a second. The training range can be conveniently set by one single button touch on top-level screen.

This work represents a knowledge fusion from the areas of human-computer interaction (HCI), mobile computing, human physiology and sports. As result the system is useful for controlled sports training as also for health exercises in a broad application range, where heart rate stands for the effort level. It can be used indoor and outdoor for general gym exercises, strength training, running, cycling, and skiing.

Best comfort is reached, when the heart monitor is not carried close to the body, but if it is mounted in best viewing distance and direction. The latter would be achieved easily by commonly available smartphone holders for bicycles and automotive. For outdoor sports without machines like running and walking, certainly the current system is sensed as not being optimal due to its size and weight; some concept additions would be required to improve it. In particular, development work was started already for coupling smart watches as primary display unit to the core HR monitoring system that is running on the smartphone. Furthermore, a broader feedback from friendly user tests certainly will lead to additional detail improvements.

Already now – also in comparison to recent consumer market products – the heart rate monitor, which was developed here, is funded on appropriate and modern HCI concepts and it will by that ease the control of sports activities for achieving in the end the desired training results more efficiently.

References

1. Kindermann, W., Simon, G., Keul, J.: The significance of the aerobic-anaerobic transition for the determination of work load intensities during endurance training. Eur. J. Appl. Physiol. **42**, 25–34 (1979)
2. Arts, F.J., Kuipers, H.: The relation between power output, oxygen uptake and heart rate in male athletes. Int. J. Sports Med. **15**(5), 228–231 (1994)
3. Hoppeler, H., Howald, H., Conley, K., Lindstedt, S.L., Claassen, H., Vock, P., Weibel, E.R.: Endurance training in humans: aerobic capacity and structure of skeletal muscle. J. Appl. Physiol. **59**(2), 320–327 (1985)
4. Tabata, I., Nishimura, K., Kouzaki, M., Hirai, Y., Ogita, F., Miyachi, M., Yamamoto, K.: Effects of moderate-intensity endurance and high-intensity intermittent training on anaerobic capacity and $VO2_{max}$. Med. Sci. Sports Exerc. **28**(10), 1327–1330 (1996)
5. Weghorn, H.: Applying mobile phone technology for making health and rehabilitation monitoring more affordable. In: Biosignals and Biorobotics Conference (BRC), 2013 ISSNIP, Rio de Janeiro, Brazil, pp. 1–5 (2013)
6. Brown, M.B.: Human-Computer Interface Design Guidelines, Chapter Four "Color", pp. 66–79. Intellect Books Ltd., Exeter (1999)
7. Kiefer, R.J., Angell, L.S.: A comparison of the effects of an analog versus digital speedometer on driver performance in a task environment similar to driving. J. Vis. Veh. **4**, 283–290 (1993)

8. Carter, R.C.: Visual search with color. J. Exp. Psychol. Hum. Percept. Perform. **8**(1), 127–136 (1982)
9. Robertson, P.K.: Visualizing color gamuts: a user interface for the effective use of perceptual color spaces in data displays. IEEE Comput. Gr. Appl. **8**(5), 50–64 (1988)
10. Dynastream Innovations Inc.: ANT message protocol and usage, Rev. 4.5 (2011). http://thisisant.com
11. Josenhans, W.T.: Breath holding effects on ULF displacement ballistocardiography. Bibl. Cardiol. **19**, 49–62 (1967)
12. Collins, C., Galpin, M., Kaeppler, M.: Android in Practice. Manning Publications, Westampton (2011)
13. Android Open Source Project.: Bluetooth low energy (2013). http://developer.android.com//guide/topics/connectivity/bluetooth-le.html. Accessed 9 May 2014
14. Dynastream Innovations Inc.: ANT+/BT smart comparison (2014). http://thisisant.com/developer/ant-plus/ant-ble-comparison. Accessed 9 May 2014
15. Dawson, E.A., Shave, R., George, K., Whyte, G., Ball, D., Gaze, D., Collinson, P.: Cardiac drift during prolonged exercise with echocardiographic evidence of reduced diastolic function of the heart. Eur. J. Appl. Psychol. **94**(3), 305–309 (2005)

Modelling Peloton Dynamics in Competitive Cycling: A Quantitative Approach

Erick Martins Ratamero$^{(\boxtimes)}$

MOAC Doctoral Training Centre, University of Warwick,
Gibbet Hill Road, Coventry CV4 7AL, UK
e.martins-ratamero@warwick.ac.uk

Abstract. We propose an agent-based model for peloton dynamics in competitive cycling. It aims to generate the very complex behaviour observed in real-life competitive cycling from a collection of agents with simple rules of behaviour. Cyclists in a peloton try to minimize their energy expenditure by riding behind other cyclists, in areas of reduced air resistance. Drafting cyclists spend considerably less energy than frontrunners, making the strategies in the sport to be based around trailing as much as possible. We quantify energy expenditure and recovery in relation to cyclists' positions in the peloton. Finally, we analyse the results and try to compare them to real-life behaviour of competitive pelotons.

Keywords: Agent-based modelling · Computer simulation · Peloton dynamics · Flocking · Emerging complexity

1 Introduction

Despite the appearance of a purely individual sport where the strongest tends to win, there is a very deep tactical layer to competitive cycling. A very simple fact generates complex behaviours and strategies: the fact that air resistance dominates the energy expenditure of athletes. The drafting effect, thus, plays a big role on peloton dynamics. The existence of a peloton itself can be explained by this effect: energy expenditure when drafting in a single line is reduced by approximately 18 % at 32 km/h, 27 % at 40 km/h, when drafting a single rider, and by as much as 39 % at 40 km/h in a group of eight riders [1].

From this fact, the behaviour observed in a real-life cycling race emerges: riders tend to group together and rotate in front of the peloton, trying to minimize the average energy expenditure of the group. When someone tries to break away from the pack of riders, the peloton decides either to chase them or let them open a time gap. If the group is deemed too dangerous, the typical behaviour is to chase it, and by having a bigger number of athletes to share the time spent in non-drafting positions, they normally succeed in this task. Only when a breakaway group is considered harmless enough a gap is established, and the tired riders from this group are normally caught close to the finish line.

Based on contributions [2,3], we take a mathematical approach trying to quantify energy expenditures based on different factors as speed, gradient of the

© Springer International Publishing Switzerland 2015
J. Cabri et al. (Eds.): icSPORTS 2013, CCIS 464, pp. 42–56, 2015.
DOI: 10.1007/978-3-319-17548-5_4

terrain, cross-section area and weight of the cyclist, and specific physiological characteristics of each individual. We regard the rider basically as a static engine on the bike, and consider the external factors that try to impede motion, such as drag resistance, rolling resistance and changes in the potential energy (such as when climbing a hill). Based on these opposing forces and in physiological data from professional cyclists, we establish an energy balance consistent with real-life values.

This is not the first agent-based approach for modelling competitive cycling; another work [3] does this, albeit with a different approach and with different goals. Their work has a focus on final results of a race and a game-theoretical, best-response model for elaborating strategies; it does not concern itself with peloton dynamics, nor with the relationship between those and the energy expenditures. In this work, we focus not on the actual results of a race, but rather on simulating the behaviour of a peloton during a race, under different circumstances.

Here, we take the peloton as a complex dynamical system. We establish general principles and rules for the behaviour of each agent, roughly based on flocking models already existing [4], calculating cohesive and separating forces for each agent, so that they stay together as a group, but having spatial gaps between them. We alter this model so that it makes sense in the context of this work and observe a self-organizing pattern emerge, resembling other natural dynamical systems [5].

We develop a model proposal for the dynamic behaviour of a competitive cycling peloton, in an agent-based fashion, based on a small set of basic rules for each agent. This rules are derived from the mathematical, physiological and dynamical concepts presented, and the emerging patterns are roughly similar to those observed in real life and in other systems.

Finally, we discuss the results based on data generated during simulations for many different parameters of the system. Starting from this data, we try to establish similarities with real-life cycling behaviour and validate the constructed model. We see this work as a first step to possible further analysis of this sport via computational simulation in the future, integrating even more parameters for natural influence and specific behaviour of the agents, based on further empirical data.

2   The Model

When constructing our model, we search for different kinds of parameters in order to replicate and extend the real-life behaviour of cyclists in a peloton. This work proposes an agent-based model for that. Agent-based models are very well suited for situations where dynamics emerge from simple interactions between different individuals, or agents [6].

2.1   Dynamical Parameters

In this section, we describe the utilized dynamical parameters for our model; that is, the set of parameters responsible for interaction between agents and the peloton behaviour. This is a central part in our model. A non-desirable choice of values here leads to unordered behaviour from the agents, rendering our energy balance equations completely useless and turning the model away from the dynamics it expects to simulate.

As a starting point for our dynamics, we take a simple flocking model [4]. In this model, agents are subject to three different kinds of forces: separating, aligning and cohesive forces. The separating force is intended to make agents keep a minimum separation between them, so that they do not collapse to a single point. This is well-suited to our model, since cyclists will try to steer away from other fellow cyclists, to avoid crashes.

In the original flocking model we have, then, an aligning force. This force is applied to each agent to make it follow the direction of their nearest neighbours. In our case, this seems a bit out of place. Naturally, in a bicycle race, all competitors are following the same direction, and steering inside the peloton is a relatively small change in direction. This way, we have decided to model intra-peloton movement purely by lateral movement, without change of heading direction. There is no need, then, for an aligning force.

Finally, we have a cohesion force. In the flocking model, each agent turns in to become closer to its mates, making the group coherent. As we want to simulate a peloton behaviour, it makes sense to apply this kind of force in our model.

In the original model, the resulting behaviour of the agents is to move around freely when far from other agents. However, when approaching other agents, this group tends to become a coherent flock, with agents exhibiting similar headings and staying together, but with some spatial separation between them.

As an improvement on this flocking model, we take the Swarm Chemistry model [7]. This time, different sets of agents have different parameters for cohesive, separating and alignment forces, making the proportion between those different, as it can be seen in Algorithm 1 (Fig. 1). This makes different sets behave in different ways, and they tend to stay together in space, even though they are not coupled together by anything other than the similarity of their parameters.

Algorithm 1 Sayama's algorithm for cohesive and separating forces

for $i \in agents$ **do**
  $N \leftarrow \{j \neq i, |x_i - x_j| < R_i\}$
  if $N \neq 0$ **then**
    $\langle x \rangle \leftarrow \sum_j \frac{x_j}{|N|}$
    $a \leftarrow c_1^i(\langle x \rangle - x_i) + c_3^i \sum_j (\frac{x_i - x_j}{|x_i - x_j|^2})$
  end if
end for

Fig. 1. Sayama's algorithm for cohesive and separating forces.

We take the way of calculating separating and cohesive forces, with minor adjustments, from this model. We calculate an acceleration for each agent, based on its relative position to the others. However, this code calculates it taking into account any other agent inside R_i, a vision radius. This way, vision is isotropic. As we are trying to model human behaviour, it is useful to tweak this so that we only take into account agents that could possibly be seen by a human, that is, contained inside a visual cone. We also want to take different scales of distance when calculating cohesive and separating forces. Cohesive force should be a long-range calculation, taking into account pretty much any other agent in the visual field, while separating forces should be more local, with only close agents being taken into account.

Based on these assumptions, we present the pseudo-code for these forces, defined here as Algorithm 2 (Fig. 2).

Algorithm 2 MOPED's algorithm for cohesive and separating forces

---

    for $i \in agents$ **do**
      $N_c \leftarrow \{j \neq i, x_j \in C_i^c\}$
      $N_s \leftarrow \{l \neq i, x_l \in C_i^s\}$
      if $N_c \neq 0$ **then**
        $\langle x \rangle \leftarrow \sum_j \frac{x_j}{|N|}$
        $a_c \leftarrow c_1^i(\langle x \rangle - x_i)$
        $a_s \leftarrow c_3^i \sum_l (\frac{x_i - x_l}{|x_i - x_l|^2})$
        $a \leftarrow a_c + a_s$
      end if
    end for

Fig. 2. MOPEDs algorithm for cohesive and separating forces.

In Algorithm 2 (Fig. 2), N_c and N_s are, respectively, the neighbourhoods used for the calculation of cohesive and separating forces. These neighbourhoods are cones with an aperture angle of $140°$, defined to mimic a human visual cone, and different radii. The neighbourhood for cohesive force is being used with a radius of 20 m, and the separating one with a radius of 2 m, so that the rider only tries to avoid contact with other agents in the immediate neighbourhood.

A last point to be addressed in this section is some kind of bias to the center; real cyclists tend to be as close to the center of the road as possible in the case where no wind is blowing, so as to avoid danger on the fringes of the road. For that, a very small bias is put in place. Also, as in any flocking model, a small, random acceleration is put into place.

As a final addendum, we introduce the concept of *active* riders: a rider is considered active if he is willing to cooperate and be the frontrunner of the peloton, being out of drafting positions in order to protect the other cyclists. This is modelled by adding a small bias to the front for active cyclists, as far as they are not already the frontrunners.

Fig. 3. View of a simulation of the peloton.

We observe that this algorithm, with the right set of parameters, yields a very life-like behaviour, with a narrow peloton front giving place to a wider formation behind, as it can be seen at Fig. 3.

2.2 Energetic Parameters

We will now group together mechanical and physiological parameters, since both sets of parameters affect the energetic balance of the cyclist, making it easier to analyse them together.

Physiological data about cyclists is abundant; the literature on how the human body behaves under these circumstances is extensive and it is not our idea to redefine anything on this domain, but rather to use existing results and adjust our model to reflect them.

Many mathematical models for competitive cycling exist already. For this model, we will use elements from Olds [2], who has a validated, well-behaved set of equations for energy expenditures. We also use specific results from Hoenigman et al. [3], who extended Olds' results and applied it on an agent-based model, and Martin et al. [8] for the potential-energy equation. By taking an agent-based approach and simulating both peloton dynamics and energy expenditures, we believe it is possible to have a more complete model and simulations that yield results that are closer to real life.

Our first point is to calculate the drafting coefficient, that is, a correction factor relating the air resistance when drafting and when not drafting. Kyle [9] measured this coefficient experimentally and affirms that the reduction in air resistance diminishes when wheel spacing increases. This is a fairly intuitive result. He mentions that this reduction obeyed a second-order polynomial, but he does not present the equation. Olds [2] reconstructs the equation from the graphical data, arriving at

$$CF_{draft} = 0.62 - 0.0104d_w + 0.0452d_w^2 \qquad (1)$$

where d_w is the wheel spacing (in meters) between the bicycle and the preceding rider, and CF_{draft} is the correction coefficient. However, Eq. 1 can be applied only when drafting happens in a paceline, that is, when riders are exactly behind one another. In a peloton, drafting occur also in other ways; riders in a diagonal have a "comet's tail" effect, with drafting bonuses decreasing when the rider behind moves backwards or sideways. There is no extensive study of drafting coefficients when a cyclist is not directly behind another one, as there is scarce data about drafting multiple riders; we only know for sure that drafting behind multiple riders is more beneficial than behind only one [1]. In this situation, we have decided to assign weights depending on the angle of view to the preceding rider. It is important to notice that drafting benefits are negligible in a distance over 3m, and therefore we limit our calculations to this radius.

Having calculated CF_{draft}, we can now go on to the power equations. As we are using a scale of one iteration per second of simulation, there is no need to account for the difference between power and energy: they are numerically the same. From Hoenigman et al. [3], we have the following equations:

$$P_{air} = kCF_{draft}v^3 \tag{2}$$

$$P_{roll} = C_r g(M + Mb)v \tag{3}$$

On Eq. 2, k is a lumped constant for aerodynamic drag, dependant, between other things, on the cross-section area of the cyclist. This constant is generally reported with the value 0.185 kg/m, and we are following this value. Of course, v is wind speed (and, as we are considering only a situation without wind, is equal to ground speed). On Eq. 3, C_r is a lumped constant for all frictional losses on a bike, and is generally reported with a value of 0.0053. Of course, g is the usual gravitational constant (9.81 m/s^2). The variables M and M_b represent, respectively, the mass of the cyclist and of the bicycle. On this model, we are using values of 63 kg and 7 kg, respectively, for these variables, without any variation between cyclists.

These equations are enough for modelling the energy expenditure of a cyclist in a flat, non-windy situation. However, we want to model also the behaviour of the peloton in uphills and downhills, and therefore we need an extra equation for that. Martin et al. [8] present this equation, for grades up to 10 % (where we consider $\sin(\arctan(G_r)) = G_r$):

$$P_{PE} = G_r g(M + Mb)v \tag{4}$$

and, therefore, we can introduce this on Eq. 3, obtaining the following:

$$P_{roll+PE} = (C_r + G_r)g(M + Mb)v \tag{5}$$

and a total energy expense of:

$$P_t = E_t = (C_r + G_r)g(M + Mb)v + kCF_{draft}v^3 \tag{6}$$

But this is only taking into account the energy expenditure. We need to model how the cyclists react to this and how much energy they can spend without exhausting themselves. For that, we will introduce the concept of lactate or anaerobic threshold, very well-known in any endurance sport. Roughly speaking, the lactate threshold is the power output an athlete is capable of without accumulating lactic acid in his muscles, that is, without getting tired [10]. In this model, we will assess how tired a rider is through a simple "energy-left" variable, so that, at lactate threshold, the value of this variable is roughly unchanged.

As presented in Hoenigman et al. [3], a speed of $0.7S_m$ is slightly under the lactate threshold, where S_m is the speed at which a rider can travel at his Max_{10} power output. The Max_{10} represents the 10-minute maximum power a rider can generate, and is generally regarded as an indicator of a rider's skill level. We are using, as in that work, a mean value for Max_{10} $\mu = 7.1\,\mathrm{W/kg}$. That represents, for a rider with 63 kg, a Max_{10} of approximately 450 W. This is equivalent, on flat ground, to $S_m = 12.96\,\mathrm{m/s}$. Therefore, $0.7S_m$ is approximately 9 m/s, and this should be slightly under lactate threshold. Finally, we take 10 m/s as a representative value for this threshold, and set a "recovery" variable, normally distributed with $\mu = 225\,\mathrm{W}$, that will be deduced from the actual spent energy. Only an energy expenditure over this limit will make the rider grow tired.

We are still faced with the challenge of determining how long does it take for a rider over his anaerobic threshold to be exhausted. For that, we will use the concept of time to exhaustion (T_{lim}), as defined in Olds [2]. The defining equation for T_{lim} is

$$\ln(T_{lim}) = -6.351 \ln(fVO_{2_{max}}) + 2.478 \tag{7}$$

In this equation, $fVO_{2_{max}}$ is the fraction of the $VO_{2_{max}}$ (maximum oxygen consumption) being used. We can substitute that for Max_{10} generating then:

$$\ln(T_{lim}) = -6.351 \ln(\frac{P_{tot}}{Max_{10}}) + 2.478 \tag{8}$$

For establishing which would be the initial value of "energy-left" to each rider, we decided to take an average situation: a sole rider at 45 km/h (or 12 m/s). From that, with our typical Max_{10} of 450 W, we calculate which would be the time to exhaustion. From there, considering our average recovery of 225 W, we calculated how much reserves a cyclist should have at the beginning of the simulation to achieve this typical time to exhaustion.

2.3 An Overview of the Model

We have presented the two parts of the model: the dynamical parameters and equations and the energetic parameters and equations. Now, we present how these two parts are interconnected.

It is clear that the position of an athlete inside the peloton greatly affects his energy balance: if a rider spends the whole time in front of the peloton, he should use more energy than another one sitting safely behind another cyclist. This way, the dynamical parameters and equations are influential on the energy balance. On the other hand, in our model, the energy balance is, usually, not relevant for the positioning of the cyclist: position calculation depends only on neighbouring agents. However, when the cyclist becomes tired, this is relevant to his position. We have postulated that a rider with less than 100 kJ of energy left is declared "exhausted". An exhausted rider has a backward bias and is effectively slower than the peloton average. This way, he tends to hang at the back of the peloton,

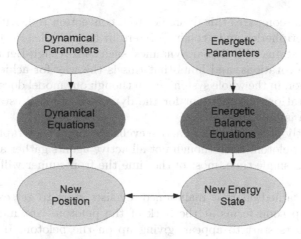

Fig. 4. Schematic diagram showing the relation between parts of the model.

eventually letting the group go altogether. A rider with 0 energy left quits the peloton altogether. In our model, he is positioned in the leftmost coordinate and becomes even slower. However, if he can somehow recover energy enough to get out of this condition altogether, he will rejoin the peloton. We present Fig. 4, a small, schematic flowchart representing the relation between the two "sides" of our model.

3   Results

In the following section, we summarize the results obtained from the simulations using MOPED. These are divided between general behaviour, dynamical and energetic results, for clarity purposes.

3.1   General Behaviour

In general, the emerging complex behaviour from the agents is very promising; riders rotate back when they feel they are under the average energy of the peloton. The peloton itself conforms to the general form of real-life pelotons, with a very narrow front (usually a 3–5 long single line of riders) and a widening profile as we look backwards.

We rapidly see a convection dynamic settling in. Riders at the back of the peloton wishing to move forwards take the sides to do that, since the middle is cluttered with cyclists and going through is virtually impossible. When they get to the front, they normally settle down in the center of the road, and as they stay there other riders coming from the back start to overtake them. This way, we have forward-moving cyclists taking the sides, backward-moving cyclists staying in the middle. Of course, to move forwards through the sides, the athletes end up spending more energy than those in the center of the peloton.

Trenchard [5] compares this dynamics to a convection roll, with "warming" riders in the peripheries and "cooling" riders in the middle. He then presents other natural systems with similar dynamics, such as Rayleigh-Bernard cells and penguin huddle rotations, and hints that this is the way for achieving optimal energy dissipation in the whole system. Even though our model does not take any energy considerations into account for the dynamics, we still establish similar patterns, which is quite interesting.

Independently of the number of active cyclists chosen, they rapidly take over the head of the peloton. Even though not all active agents gather at the front of the peloton at a single time, most of the time the frontrunner will be an active cyclist.

When a sustained effort is maintained, cyclists start to get exhausted and a sizeable group soon forms at the back of the peloton. Not much after, the first spent cyclists start to appear, giving up on the peloton. If this effort is maintained for long enough, only the strongest riders stay in the peloton, with all the rest giving up. This is consistent with long climbs in professional races, where the front group is normally smaller than ten cyclists. Also as in real life cycling, a long descent after a climb has the effect of bringing lots of cyclists back to the peloton, as they recover energy.

3.2 Dynamical Parameters

Most of the results about the dynamics are difficult to quantify. As commented in the section above, the general behaviour of the peloton seems coherent with real life and, furthermore, coherent with an optimal energy dissipation.

As an addendum, we can show graphically the convection dynamics. On Fig. 5, we have a graph of average draft coefficient for agents moving forwards (blue) and backwards (red). It is clear that, on average, forwards-moving cyclists on the periphery will have less opportunities to draft behind another cyclists, and the opposite happens with the central, backwards-moving agents.

3.3 Energetic Parameters

At first, for illustrating which kind of behaviour our model generates, we start with an example. We submit 100 agents to a 3-hour race at a constant speed of 45 km/h. Of course this speed is too high for uphill parts, making them spend much more energy than humanly possible, but we are only interested in the qualitative behaviour that exhaustion generates. We generate a profile for the race, plotting the elevation at each time. As we are at constant speed, it is the same as plotting elevation per distance. The generated profile is represented on Fig. 6. Subjecting our cyclists to this profile, we generate, then, a graph illustrating the amount of exhausted riders at any given time. The plot is shown as Fig. 7.

We can now establish correlations between both plots. In the very long initial uphill, relatively few riders were exhausted. That is, of course, because at the beginning of the race, every athlete is still fresh. A slight downhill follows, enough

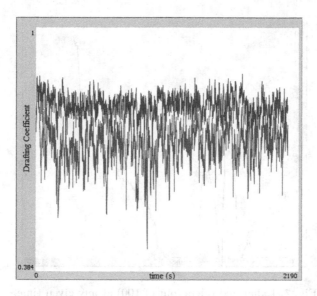

Fig. 5. Temporal distribution of draft coefficient for backward and forward-moving agents.

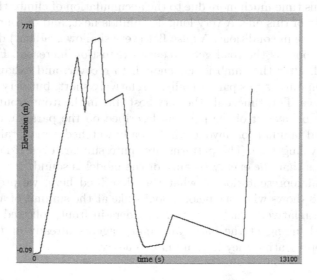

Fig. 6. Temporal profile of our test race.

to recover all cyclists. However, a second, steepest uphill follows, and this time the exhaustion is much bigger in the peloton. Even during the shallow part close to the summit, the number of exhausted riders is still increasing considerably. Another downhill follows and, again, it is enough to recover all riders. Now, a short, not too steep climb is presented, and the result is a big increase again in

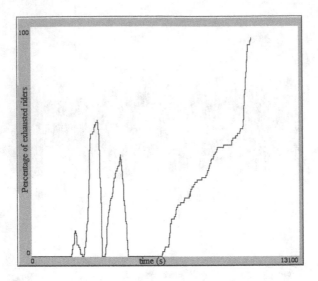

Fig. 7. Exhausted riders (out of 100) at any given time.

exhaustion, this time much more due to the accumulation of climbs than because of the difficulty of this one. A very long downhill is next, and of course all riders arrive down there in conditions. A false-flat (very shallow gradient) do not break them, but as soon as the road gets steeper exhaustion increases. Even a long, slight downhill after the climb is not enough to recover, and exhaustion keeps increasing even during this part. Finally, a relatively short, but very steep climb to finish the race. This time, only the very best stay in the front group at the top.

The whole behaviour of the peloton described on the paragraph above will certainly sound familiar for anyone who already watched a mountain stage in a professional cycling race. The patterns are quite similar, even if not identical, which indicates that the energy balance of the model is sound.

As a visual representation of what was described here, we present Figs. 8 and 9. Figure 8 shows what the peloton looks like at the summit of a long climb. You can see a relatively small group of 14 riders in front, followed by a bigger group barely hanging at the back, and many agents already at the leftmost coordinate, representing they have no more energy.

Fig. 8. Peloton at the top of a climb.

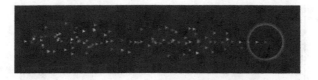

Fig. 9. Peloton during the descent.

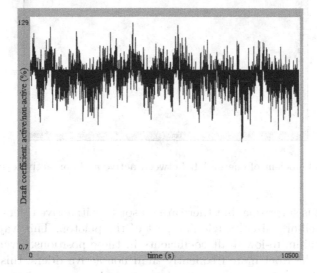

Fig. 10. Draft coefficient of active riders, as a percentage of DC of non-active riders.

As a comparison, Fig. 9 shows the peloton during the descent, when the lesser riders have already recovered. You can see the peloton shape is still longest than normal due to the fact that the back riders are still coming back, but there are no more riders with no energy left and the group is unified again.

Finally, we present an interesting, counter-intuitive result derived from the model. We start by drawing, at Fig. 10, the average draft coefficient for active riders (considering 20 out 100 to be active riders) compared to the average draft coefficient of non-active ones.

The horizontal reference level is 100 %, which would mean that, on average, active and non-active riders have similar draft coefficients. However, that is not what the graph shows: even if it is not that easy to see on this plot, active riders have lower draft coefficients on average, which means they spend less energy. To confirm that, we plot a quocient between average energy for active and non-active cyclists, and, even though it starts at 1 as expected, it undoubtedly increases with time, indicating active riders are, indeed, spending less energy on average. This plot is presented as Fig. 11.

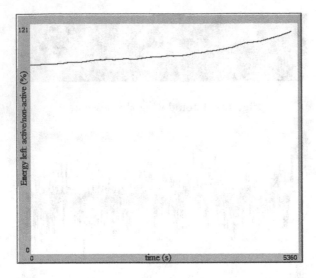

Fig. 11. Quocient of energy left between active and non-active cyclists.

This result is surprising, but there are reasons for it: active riders spend more time on the well-organized, single line part of the peloton. This way, they have constantly medium-to-low draft coefficients in these positions. Even if they do have to go to the front more frequently than non-active riders, this if offset by the fact that they are consistently drafting some other cyclists. Non-active riders spend more time in the convection-like part of the peloton, constantly going back and forth and spending considerable amount of time in non-drafting positions at the periphery of the peloton. Furthermore, if we can imagine the speed of a cyclist as an oscillatory function around the average speed of the peloton (with the oscillations being in the periods where the cyclist move forwards or backwards), cyclists in the peloton have a bigger oscillatory amplitude than active ones. As the air resistance scales with the third power of speed, this by itself would cause a bigger air resistance.

Besides that, with much more movement inside the peloton, they are not guaranteed to have another rider right in front of them at all times, as someone in the single-line part of the peloton does. This way, their draft coefficient is much more subject to variations.

This can also be shown by Fig. 12, where we plot a quocient between average neighbourhood size for active and non-active agents. At the beginning, when the active agents are still organizing themselves, the plot goes under and over 1, but it quickly settles under 1 as soon as the active riders organize themselves. This shows that they are getting smaller draft coefficients in spite of drafting less cyclists, which is coherent with the idea that they spend more time exactly behind another cyclist.

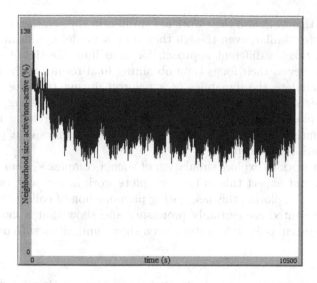

Fig. 12. Average size of active-agent neighborhood compared to nonactive agents.

4   Discussion

This work presents a model for peloton dynamics in competitive cycling, using an agent-based approach. Based on a few simple rules for dynamics and energy balance, we derived a rather complex pattern of convection in the peloton, and coherent results in terms of energy. Some interesting, counter-intuitive results arise from the proposed model.

The result where active cyclists spent less energy than non-active ones does not conform to general knowledge in cycling, There is, however, room for improvement and calibration in the model. For instance, when moving around, agents do not look for favourable positions in terms of drafting possibilities, and the lack of data for drafting in diagonal positions and behind multiple cyclists hinder the accuracy of energy distributions.

Besides that, we do not account for many real-life factors that affect competitive cyclists. An example is wind, a factor that has major impact in many professional races. Frontal wind can be modelled as a difference in speed for the aerodynamical factor in our energy expenditure equation, but sidewinds require a whole new approach that was not within the scope of this work. Of course, there is a different dimension of cycling that was also not modelled here: the strategic part. "Intelligent" agents, who know what their best response to the circumstances of a race is, could create breakaways, become active or non-active mid-way during a race, save as much energy as possible for a final sprint. This is certainly feasible as a future model.

This is probably the first time an agent-based approach is used to try and simulate large-scale cycling peloton dynamics. Another work [3] take a similar approach, using an agent-based model to simulate results of cycling races. Many ideas between this work and their work are similar; in special, the energy balance is probably quite similar, even though they do not model uphills and downhills and this work takes a different approach for modelling the time to exhaustion of a cyclist. However, their focus is on obtaining final results of the races, while we want to simulate the dynamics of a peloton during the race. A different work [5] makes some proto-simulations of pelotons with drafting, looking for hysteresis on phase transitions. In spite of presenting interesting results, this model is not interested in simulating the complex dynamics of a peloton, but only in illustrating a concept.

As the first work to explore simulation of such a complex system as a cycling peloton, we do not expect this to be a complete work in any way, but rather to be a first step on exploring this fascinating phenomenon of collective behaviour. The results presented are certainly promising and show that a more complete model of this system is feasible and can even show similarities with other natural systems.

Acknowledgements. Many thanks to Prof. René Doursat (Institut des Systèmes Complexes Paris Île-de-France) for the teachings about agent-based models and for supporting his students' ideas. Thanks to James Newling, for the insightful discussions during the development of the model. This work was supported by an Erasmus Mundus Masters scholarship for the Complex Systems Science program.

References

1. McCole, S., Claney, K., Conte, J.C., Anderson, R., Hagberg, J.: Energy expenditure during bicycling. J. Appl. Physiol **68**, 748–753 (1990)
2. Olds, T.: The mathematics of breaking away and chasing in cycling. Eur. J. Appl. Physiol. **77**, 492–497 (1998)
3. Hoenigman, R., Bradley, E., Lim, A.: Cooperation in bike racing when to work together and when to go it alone. Complexity **17**, 39–44 (2011)
4. Wilensky, U.: NetLogo flocking model. Center for Connected Learning and Computer-Based Modeling. Northwestern University, Evanston, IL (1998)
5. Trenchard, H.: The complex dynamics of bicycle pelotons (2012). arXiv preprint arXiv:1206.0816
6. Woolridge, M.: Introduction to Multiagent Systems. John Wiley & Sons, New York (2001)
7. Sayama, H.: Decentralized control and interactive design methods for large-scale heterogeneous self-organizing swarms. In: Almeida e Costa, F., Rocha, L.M., Costa, E., Harvey, I., Coutinho, A. (eds.) ECAL 2007. LNCS (LNAI), vol. 4648, pp. 675–684. Springer, Heidelberg (2007)
8. Martin, J.C., Milliken, D.L., Cobb, J.E., McFadden, K.L., Coggan, A.R.: Validation of a mathematical model for road cycling power. J. Biomech. **14**, 276–291 (1998)
9. Kyle, C.R.: Reduction of wind resistance and power output of racing cyclists and runners travelling in groups. Ergonomics **22**, 387–397 (1979)
10. Vogt, S., Heinrich, L., Schumacher, Y.O., Blum, A., Roecker, K., Dickhuth, H., Schmid, A.: Power output during stage racing in professional road cycling. Med. Sci. Sports Exerc. **38**, 147–151 (2006)

Analyzing the Sensorimotor Training Using Wireless Sensors: Studying the Effects of Balance Boards with Different Dimensions of Instability

Angelina Thiers[1]([✉]), Annett l'Orteye[2], Katja Orlowski[1],
and Thomas Schrader[1]

[1] Department of Informatics and Media,
Brandenburg University of Applied Sciences, Brandenburg, Germany
{thiers,orlowski,schrader}@fh-brandenburg.de
[2] Städtisches Klinikum Brandenburg GmbH, Akademisches Lehrkrankenhaus
der Charité, Abteilung Medizinische Schule, Brandenburg, Germany

Abstract. Over the time the popularity of the application of the sensorimotor training in the fields of prevention, therapy, rehabilitation as well as for the improvement of the athletic performance increased. Nonetheless, the impact of the training on the body is not yet fully investigated. Actually, the experiences of the physiotherapist as well as the conditions of the practice determine the therapy planning. For a more detailed look of the effects of the sensorimotor training on the body, two setups were investigated. In the first part, the behavior of two students was studied on three exercisers. Here the EMG data and the motion data were analyzed. Additionally, different tests for the investigation of the laterality of the hands and the feet were made. In the second part, the behavior of the left and the right body side was analyzed for 16 subjects. The results revealed that the major work for the maintenance of the equilibrium is done by the distal musculature. Furthermore, it was shown that there is a different behavior of the musculature at both body sides. Additionally, it has been proven that each test person had an individual behavior on the exercisers. Consequently, further investigations were needed to make general assumptions regarding the impact of the training on the body.

Keywords: Sensorimotor training · EMG data · Motion data · Wireless sensors

1 Introduction

The sensorimotor training offers a great variety of application fields as well as a lot of different exercisers. Hence, it is going to be more and more attractive. Nevertheless, the training itself is not completely investigated until now [1].

In the physiotherapists practice the training is used for prevention, therapy, rehabilitation as well as for the improvement of the athletic performance [2].

© Springer International Publishing Switzerland 2015
J. Cabri et al. (Eds.): icSPORTS 2013, CCIS 464, pp. 57–71, 2015.
DOI: 10.1007/978-3-319-17548-5_5

Firstly Dr. Vladimir Janda noticed that regarding the control of human movement there is a direct correlation of the sensory and the motor system. He pointed out that both systems react as one and that changes in one system also lead to reactions in the other system. He also introduced the term "sensorimotor system". His studies showed that the proprioception, also known as depth sensitivity, is the most significant aspect for the coordination of movement. As part of his investigations he developed the sensorimotor training [3,4].

Besides that the motor unit activity is also a keyword of the sensorimotor training. Motor unit activity comprises the terms of reflexes, controlled voluntary movements as well as rhythmic and cyclical motion patterns. The overall process of the coordination of the movement is a complex process. Consequently, the success of the training depends mostly on the correct and professional execution of the training [4].

The growing popularity of the sensorimotor training causes a huge range of different exercisers for supporting. The great amount of different exercisers and the fact that the sensorimotor training, especially the therapy planning is not fully investigated, make the execution of an effective training quite difficult.

Nowadays the application of the exercisers as well as the planning of the whole therapy is mainly based on the experiences of the physiotherapist and of the given possibilities in their practice [1]. The information about the exercisers published by the manufacturers or in the literature may have an influence on the planning of the training. For example, the Balance Board should strengthen the musculature of the buttocks, the legs, the back and the abdomen [5]. The maintenance of the equilibrium on the Balance Board should have different effects. The first effect is the improvement of the inter- and intramuscular coordination of the muscles of the feet and the legs. The second effect, staying with both feed on the Balance Board, is the enhancement of the stabilization in the region of the lumbar spine, the pelvis and the hip. The last effect is the optimization of the inter- and intramuscular coordination of muscles of the lumbar spine, the thoracic spine and the cervical spine [6]. Another example says that the beginners should use an exerciser like the Rocker Board. Rocker Boards have a one-dimensional instability. The principle behind: the higher the instability the more the musculature has to stabilize [7].

In summary there are the following problems regarding the planing of the sensorimotor training:

1. Great variety of exerciser
2. Assumption of the expected trainings effects of the exercisers are based on:
   (a) the manufactures informations
   (b) the literature
   (c) the physiotherapists knowledge
3. It is difficult to verify the expected trainings effects

For the analyzes of the sensorimotor training, especially regarding the first two items, an investigation of the effects of three different exercisers was made. Thereby two exercisers with a one-dimensional and one exerciser with an multi-dimensional instability were compared.

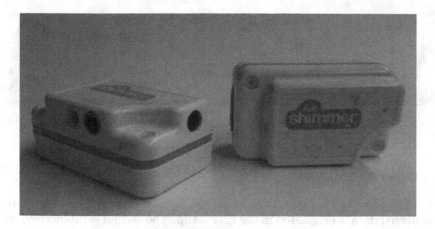

Fig. 1. Shimmer sensors.

2 Material and Methods

2.1 Measurements

The Shimmer^{TM} measuring instruments are small wireless sensors, Fig. 1. The Bluetooth technology enables to stream the data online and in real-time. The used sensors were a combination of the baseboard and different daughterboards. The used daughterboards were the electromyogram (EMG) as well as the gyroscope sensor. The dimensions are about 53 mm × 32 mm × 15 mm [8].

The EMG module allows the one channel measurement of the electrical activity of a muscle. Providing pre-amplification of EMG signal the non-invasive method represents the whole activity of a muscle [9].

The gyroscope daughterboard consists of a single and a dual axis angular rate gyroscope and is able to measure three angular velocity [10].

2.2 Exercisers

Balance Board. The Balance Board is an exerciser with a multidimensional instability, Fig. 2, which offers different fields of application. The height of the exerciser is 9 cm. The Balance Board supports the strengthening of the musculature of the buttocks, the legs, the back as well as the abdomen [5].

Rocker Board. The Rocker Board is characterized by its one-dimensional instability with a height of 7.5 cm, Fig. 2. The exerciser offers either a forward-backward or a left-right instability. The Rocker Board is made to train the coordination, the stamina, the strength as well as the motor skills [11].

The left-right deflection requires movement patterns performed by the extension and the flexion of the knee joints. In contrast, the forward-backward deflection aims for the reaction of the ankle joint.

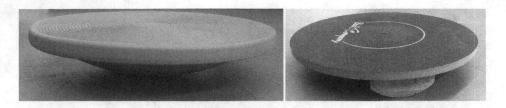

Fig. 2. Balance Board and Rocker Board.

2.3 Experimental Setups

During the investigation two different setups were analyzed. The main part of the analyzed data is originated in the first setup. The second setup derived from a previous study [12] and was added for statistical analyzes. The first setup is meant to prove the assumption that the training on the exerciser causes effects on the whole body. The aim of the second setup was the investigation of the participation of both body sides during the sensorimotor training [13].

Supporting the objective to develop a user-oriented experimental setup the design of the study was made in cooperation with experienced physiotherapists of a medical school. The requirement to develop a test procedure which can also be executed with patients causes the drop out of the maximum voluntary contraction (MVC) measurement. Instead of the MVC normalization a reference measurement in front of the exerciser took place.

Setup 1. The first setup comprised of two young (age under 30 years) and healthy students. Both subjects were not familiar with the exercisers. An equal distribution of the sexes was given.

For the investigation two different types of Shimmer^{TM} measurement units were used. A pair of gyroscope sensors were centrally placed on the different exercisers. For the verification of the assumption that the training on the exercisers has effects to the whole body the sensors were placed at five different muscles along the body. The following five muscles were recorded: the M. tibialis anterior, the M. vastus lateralis, the M. gluteus maximus, the M. erector spinae (longissimus) and the M. trapezius. All test points have been measured on the right and on the left body side. Ag/AgCl surface electrodes were applied at the skin. The skin preparation as well as the placement of the electrodes considered the recommendations of the SENIAM project [14].

The test persons had to perform the complete test sequence for each of the three exercisers. The subjects stand on both legs for the whole time. One test sequence comprised of a reference measurement in front of the exerciser with a duration of 15 s as well as of a measurement on the equipment. This part of the procedure was divided into four consecutive phases of changing difficulty, Table 1. All phases were characterized by symmetrical requirements to both body sides. All recordings have been done without shoes. The instructions and the supervision of the correct execution were made by an experienced physiotherapist.

Table 1. Setup 1 - test procedure.

Phase	Task	Duration
1	Eyes open	30 s
2	Eyes closed	30 s
3	Throwing a medicine ball	60 s
4	Eyes open	30 s

Investigations have shown that next to handedness, the laterality is important for all paired body parts [15]. Thats why, the subjects had to perform a test to characterize their laterality of the hands and feet. On the whole, six tests for the handedness and ten tests for the laterality of the feet were made. Additionally, a balance test was made, too. The task was to stand on two scales, with each foot on one scale. The distribution of the weight was documented.

Setup 2. The second setup involved 16 healthy subjects of the medical school and the university. One selection criterion was that the subjects have to be a right-hander. Two test persons of the original study were not included because their were left-hander. The test persons ranged from 20 years to 53 years in age. One half of the test persons was familiar with the used exercisers.

For the current investigation only the data of the Balance Board were analyzed. Again, different sensors were used. The skin preparation and the placement of the electrodes followed the recommendations of the SENIAM project [14].

The exercises were characterized by standing the whole time on both legs and symmetrical requirements to the body sides. In this setup one test sequence consists of a reference recording in front of the exerciser and the measurement with five different phases on the Balance Board. Four of the phases were identical to the phases of the first setup. Consequently, only these four phases were considered in the analyzes of the behavior of the left and right body side. Again, all test persons have not worn shoes.

2.4   Data Analyzes

Firstly the EMG data was notch filtered with a blocking frequency of 50 Hz. Secondly a band-pass filter was applied to the data [16]. The next step comprised the normalizations of the EMG data. The calculation of the average muscular activity when staying in front of the exerciser was used as normalization value. Subsequently, the absolute values of the measurement on the exercisers were transformed into relative values by using the normalization value. Consequently, the values were presented as percentage of the stance.

The signal processing also implies the full-wave rectification of the EMG data [16]. The evaluation of the data in the time domain includes the calculation of different statistical parameters. The maximum and mean values were computed for the whole signal over a time window of 512 ms [17]. These values were used for further calculations. On the one hand the course of the maximum values over time was documented. On the other hand the mean value of the maximum voltage values for each phase as well as for the complete procedure was calculated. Next to the mean and the maximum of the EMG the accumulated EMG activity (iEMG) was evaluated. Therefore, the EMG was integrated over time. Consequently, the total accumulated activity was computed by the calculation of the area under the EMG for a chosen time period [18,19]. This calculation was performed for each phase as well as for the complete test procedure. Furthermore, the course of the iEMG was documented by the summation of the iEMG over the time.

The transformation of the EMG signal from time into frequency domain was achieved by using the Fast Fourier Transformation over signal segments of 512 ms [20,21]. This transformation allows the computation of parameters in the frequency domain. The total power is described as the accumulation of the power density spectrum (SPD) of the whole frequencies (f), Eq. 1 [20].

$$E_{totalPower} = \int_0^\infty S_{PD}(f)df. \tag{1}$$

The parameter is used as an indicator for muscle fatigue. An increase of the total power indicates that the muscle is fatigued.

In addition to the EMG data the gyroscope data was also analyzed. The motion data was low-pass filtered. Afterwards the direction of motion as well as the current deflection was computed.

3   Results

The test for the handedness of test person one (TP 01) reveals a dominance of the right body side. In five out of six tests the right hand was the preferred one. The analysis of the test for the dominant body side of the feet shows a similar result. In seven out of ten tests the subject used the right foot. An equal distribution of the weight during the scales test was given.

The laterally test of proband two (TP 02) showed that for the verification of the handedness a preference of the right side is given. The subject solved four out of six tasks by using the right hand. Equally, the analyses of the behavior of the feet figured out that there is a dominance of the right body side. In six out of ten tests the right side was preferred. The scales balance test reveals an equal distribution of the body weight.

The accumulated EMG activity was calculated for each muscle and for each exerciser. For the comparison of the participation of the individual muscles the one with the highest activity value was declared as 100 %. All other activity values of the remaining muscles were set in relation to the 100 %.

Figure 3 shows the course of the accumulated EMG activity of the M. tibialis anterior and the M. vastus lateralis for both body sides of test person two on the left-right Rocker Board. In this case the 100 % were achieved by the right M. vastus lateralis. This observation goes along with the expected relationship of the participation of the individual muscles. The left-right Rocker Board especially requires the flexion and the extension of the knee which is among other things realized by the M. vastus lateralis.

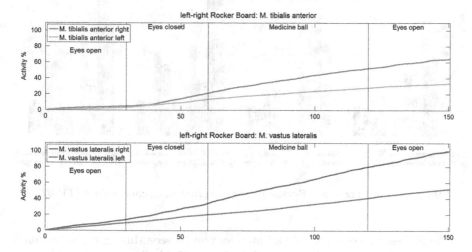

Fig. 3. Left-right rocker board - accumulated activity (TP 02).

Another outcome of Fig. 3 is that both sides of the M. tibiales anterior perform less work than the right M. vastus lateralis. It is also shown that the left muscles only carry out half of the activity compared to the right side. Additionally, it can be seen that with the beginning of the second phase the values of the EMG activity as well as the difference in the amount of the activity between the two muscles increases. Both muscles have in common that the difference in the amount of the activity level raises over time.

This behavior was analyzed in the context of the direction of motion. However the distribution of the direction does not depend on the overall time the board moved to right is similar to the overall duration of the left movements. Hence, the dominance of the right musculature depends not on the supremacy of one direction of motion. On the contrary, it goes along with the outcome of the laterality tests for the feet, where the right side was dominant.

Figure 4 visualizes the average maximum values for each phase for each muscle when test person two used the Rocker Board (left-right). The first finding is, that during the initial phase nearly for all muscles the lowest values were documented. Although, the first and the last phase require an identical task, the measured values of the last phase were higher. This highlights that there is a slow relaxation of the muscle activity.

The second finding is, that the highest values were always reached by the distal musculature. Especially, for the left and right M. gluteus maximus and the left and right M. trapezius descendens relatively low voltage values were documented.

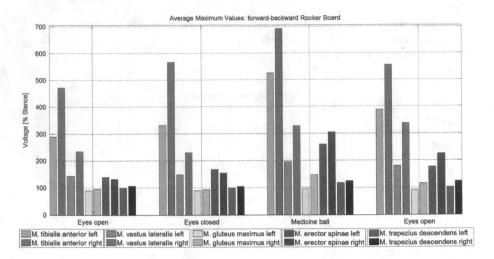

Fig. 4. Forward-backward Rocker Board - average maximum values (TP 02).

The highest values for nearly all muscles can be seen during the third phase "Medicine ball". The catching and throwing of the ball causes an additional, external stimulus which influences the maintenance of the balance. Furthermore, the execution of this motion sequence requires the left and right M. erector spinae. Consequently, for a higher participation of the back muscles an external stimulus is needed. This also supports the assumption that the major part of the work for the maintenance of the equilibrium is done by the distal musculature and that for a participation of the proximal musculature an external stimulus is required.

Another outcome of Fig. 4 is that in most cases the higher voltage values were reached by the right body side. Again, this is accompanied by the results of the laterality tests. In particular, the difference between the documented values of the left and right body side of the leg muscles supports the assumption that there is a dominance of the strain in the right body side although a symmetrical requirement to both sides is given, again.

Figure 5 shows the course of the average maximum values as well as the course of the total power of the left and right M. gluteus maximus of test person one during the usage of the Balance Board.

On the one hand the illustration points out that the right body side is generating higher voltage values over the whole time. On the other hand, it can be seen that nearly for the whole time the values of the left muscle show an amount of under 100 %. This means that the left muscle is producing lower voltage values during the measurement on the Balance Board than during the reference recording in front of the exerciser. On the contrary, the voltage values of the right M. tibialis anterior were between 200 and 2000 %. This finding is a reason to assume, that the accessory muscles, like the ischiocrural muscles, are mostly responsible for the maintenance of the functions of the M. gluteus maximus.

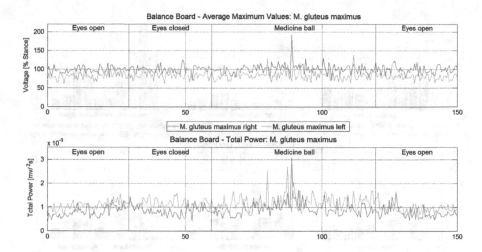

Fig. 5. Balance Board - average maximum values and total power (TP 01).

The lower section of Fig. 5 shows the course of the total power of the left and right M. gluteus maximus. Fatigue is defined in muscle physiology as a state when a subject can no longer maintain a required force [16]. Hence, the maintenance demands an increasing recruitment of motor units [22]. Although, the left M. gluteus maximus produces lower voltage values, the total power of the left muscle is nearly the whole time higher than the total power of the right body side. Consequently, the left muscle had recruited a higher number of motor units despite the lower voltage values.

The illustration 6 provides a brief overview of the complete muscular activity of each muscle on each exerciser for both test persons. The muscle with the highest strain from both subjects represents the 100 %. The values of the remaining muscles from both test persons were presented in relation to the 100 %.

The complete muscular activity for test person one for each muscle and each exerciser is documented in the upper part of the Fig. 6. The 100 % were achieved by the right M. tibiales anterior during the execution of the trial on the forward-backward Rocker Board. Furthermore, the second highest value was achieved on the same exerciser but in this case by the left M. tibialis anterior.

The figure also points out that the strain of the individual exercisers aims to different muscles. Using the Balance Board mostly burdens the left and right M. vastus lateralis. In contrast, the M. erector spinae shows for both body sides the highest values on the left-right Rocker Board. As already mentioned the forward-backward Rocker Board shows the highest strain in the M. tibialis anterior. Nevertheless, the first and last exerciser have in common, that the distal musculature shows the highest values. The ranking of the overall strain of the three exercisers shows the order (highest strain first): forward-backward Rocker Board, Balance Board, left-right Rocker Board.

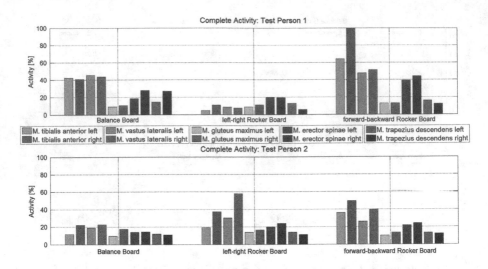

Fig. 6. Activity - comparison of the three exercisers.

The values of the complete activity of all muscles on all exercisers of test person two are presented in the lower part of Fig. 6. Test person two obtained the highest values with the right M. vastus lateralis on the left-right Rocker Board. The overall comparison of the three exercisers shows that the Balance Board seems to be the smallest challenge for the test person. In contrast, the highest complete strain was achieved by the left-right Rocker Board. The various forms of the Rocker Board required different muscles. The left-right Rocker Board has the highest effort in the right M. vastus lateralis. On the contrary, the right M. tibialis anterior shows the highest values during the usage of the forward-backward Rocker Board. Again, all exercisers have in common, that the highest values were documented for the distal musculature. The difference of the amount of the activity of the leg muscles on the individual exercisers is greater than the single values of the M. gluteus maximus, M. erector spinae and the M. trapezius descendens.

The illustration also figures out, that on each exerciser all muscles, except the M. trapezius descendens, show the highest values for the right body side. All exercisers have in common, that the EMG activity of the test person differs. Although the test persons used the same exercisers and had to handle identical tasks the individual requirements seem to be different.

The current Fig. 7 shows the deflection into the direction forward-backward. In the upper part of the figure the deflection for the Balance Board is shown. The course of the forward-backward Rocker Board is shown in the lower part of the figure.

The Balance Board shows no drift in one direction over the whole time. Only during the phase "Eyes closed" (Phase two) a drift can be seen. Immediately after the visual analyzers, the eyes, are turned on again, the drift is corrected. In the third phase greater deflections were measured, they are caused by the

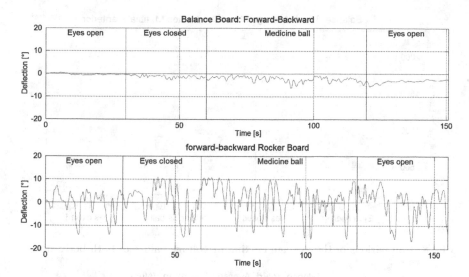

Fig. 7. Balance board and forward-backward rocker board - deviation (TP 01).

additional difficulty induced by the external stimuli of the medicine ball. On the whole, the course is characterized by small and short deflections around the baseline.

The course of the forward-backward Rocker Board only shows slight differences during the individual phases in the amount of the values of the deflection. In the first and second phase a short and small drift was documented. In both cases the drift is correct after 15/20 s. The comparison of the strength of the deflection from the forward-backward Rocker Board to the intensity of the forward-backward deflection of the Balance Board shows differences. The intensity of the deflection of the Rocker Board is much greater than the intensity of the Balance Board.

Figure 8 serves the comparison of the left-right relation of the M. tibialis anterior on the Balance Board. Therefore the average maximum voltage values of 18 test persons (two from setup one and 16 subjects from setup two) were summed up in the box plot.

The figure points out, that the highest voltage values were produced by the right M. tibialis anterior during the second phase "Eyes closed". One additional finding of the right body side during this phase is, that it has the largest range between the maximal and the minimal values. This may mean that the individual persons react in different ways to the elimination of the visual analyzer. The behavior of the test persons depend on their age, their balance skills, their muscles, their motor and coordination skills and so on. This influential factors cause, that for some people the consequences regarding the maintenance of the equilibrium are greater than for others. The Fig. 8 also brings out, that in the overview of all test persons the right side is the dominant body side for all considered scenarios. On the one hand, every time the median value is higher on

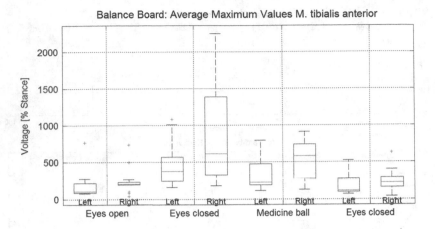

Fig. 8. Comparions of the average maximum voltage values of both body sides.

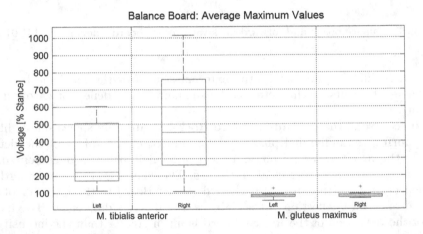

Fig. 9. Comparison of the average maximum voltage values of M. tibialis anterior and M. gluteus maximus.

the right side of the M. tibialis anterior. On the other hand, the 75 th percentile is also always greater on the right body side. In addition, the left body side has always the lowest minimum values (25 th percentiles).

The current box plot of Fig. 9 shows the average maximum voltage values of the test person from both setups for the M. tibialis anterior and the M. gluteus maximus. On the one hand the measured values again document that the major part of the work is done by the distal musculature. The median value of the M. tibialis is up to four times higher than the median value of the M. gluteus maximus. The documented values of the M. gluteus maximus correspond to the activity values during the reference measurement in front of the exerciser. Consequently, it is shown that the continuation of the muscular activity up to the proximal musculature has only a small extent because the demand to the musculature is slightly higher than in demand in front of the exerciser.

For further statistical analyzes the "Chi-squared" test was performed for the 18 test persons from setup one and setup two when using the Balance Board. The statistical investigation was made for the average maximum values for the left and right M. tibialis anterior. Therefore a comparison of the voltage values of each test person was computed. For each subject a decision which body side reached the higher values was made. The evaluation was fulfilled for each phase and for the overall measurement. Consequently, the H_0 hypothesis, that there is no dependency between the maximum values and the body side, was rejected to significance level of 5 %.

4   Discussion

The experimental study points out four important findings. Firstly, the assumption that the muscles of nearly the whole body were involved in the process of the maintenance of the equilibrium on the exercisers could not be proofed. Secondly, there is a different behavior regarding the left and right musculature. The third finding is, that it is not possible to make a general assumption, that exercisers with a one-dimensional instability are easier to handle than the exercisers with a multidimensional instability. The last finding is, that each test person shows an individual behavior on the exercisers.

The analyzes of setup one showed, that the major part of the work for the maintenance of the equilibrium is done by the distal musculature. To achieve a higher participation of the proximal musculature an external stimuli, like catching and throwing of a medicine ball is needed. Especially, for the left and right M. gluteus maximus low voltage values were documented. This observation leads to the hypothesis that the ischiocrural musculature takes the job of the M. gluteus maximus to take part in the progress of the maintenance of equilibrium.

The study of the voltage values of the left and right body side was carried out for both setups. The investigation of setup one showed that in most cases the right musculature achieved the higher voltage values. In particular, the distal musculature of the left and right body side often shows great differences between the maximum voltage values as well as between the accumulated EMG activity. This finding was supported by the statistical analyzes of the maximum voltage values for subjects of setup one and two.

Both, the EMG data and the motion data of the three exercisers, showed, that it is not possible to determine the difficulty of an exerciser by one- or multidimensional instability. The exercisers with the one-dimensional instability were in both cases the one with the greater deflection and the greater voltage values. However, both test persons from setup one achieved the highest values on different Rocker Boards.

The overall finding is, that it is not possible to make general assumptions about the usage as well as about the effects of the exercisers. This is due to the fact that the test persons showed an individual behavior on the equipment.

5   Conclusions

The investigation of the three exercisers reveals that it is necessary to analyze the sensorimotor training more detailed. It is not enough to take the manufactures information, the literature as well as the practical knowledge in consideration. Rather the results show that the application and the corresponding effects of the exercisers depend on the behavior of the subject. One solution for the improvement and the verification of the training is the application of wireless sensors. The usage of wireless sensors is a helpful instrument to analyze the behavior of different subjects on the exercisers. Consequently, the physiotherapist has to consider the characteristics of the patient in the planning of the therapy. Furthermore, the use of wireless sensors are a very good way to document the development and the results of the therapy. The physiotherapist are able to control the changes of the behavior of the muscles.

A second point for an effective planning of the therapy is excellent knowledge about the exerciser. In the majority of cases the product descriptions include information of the material, the height, the diameter and sometimes the angle of deflection. All analyzed exercisers have similar values regarding the height, the diameter as well as the angle of deflection. Nevertheless, the test persons showed different activation patterns. This leads to the recommendation that the product descriptions should include additional information, for example about the own weight of the exerciser or information about the special characteristics of the supporting surface.

The current results can be extended to more detailed analyzes of the behavior of the muscles in dependency of the movement on the exerciser and with a greater number of test persons. With the help of the mobile sensors it is also possible to give an immediate feedback for the correction of the dominance of one body side. This different behavior of the body sides will be analyzed more detailed in further studies. In this context we will also analyze whether the dominance of the right side is caused by the fact that the test persons were all right handed.

References

1. Rühl, J., Laubach, V.: Funktionelles Zirkeltraining: Das moderne Sensomotoriktraining für alle. Meyer & Meyer Verlag, Aachen (2012)
2. Häfelinger, U., Schuba, V.: Koordinationstherapie: Propriozeptives Training. Meyer & Meyer Verlag, Aachen (2010)
3. Page, P.: Sensorimotor training: a global approach for balance training. J. Bodywork Mov. Ther. **10**(1), 77–84 (2005)
4. Lukas, C., Fröhlich, V., Kapferer, H., Zelder, C.: Sprunggelenksverletzungen im Basketball: Hintergründe, Therapie und Prophylaxe. Books on Demand, Birmingham (2011)
5. Sport-Thieme®: Sport- und Therapiekreisel, http://www.webcitation.org/6Bgic Ok7Y
6. Bertram, A.M., Laube, W.: Sensomotorische Koordination: Gleichgewichtstraining auf dem Kreisel. Thieme, Stuttgart (2008)

7. Grifka, J., Dullien, S.: Knie und Sport: Empfehlungen von Sportarten aus orthopädischer und sportwissenschaftlicher Sicht. Deutscher Arzte-Verlag, cologne (2008)
8. Shimmer Research: Shimmer-Brochure-Pack (2011)
9. Shimmer Research Support: EMG User Guide Rev 1.2 (2012)
10. Kuris, B.: Kinematics Guide Revision 1e (2010)
11. Bad-Company: Deluxe Balance Board Set 45 cm aus Holz in Studio-Qualität, http://www.webcitation.org/6Fg4kjCXJ
12. Thiers, A., Meffofok, L., Orlowski, K., Schrader, K., Titze, B., l'Orteye, A., Schrader, T.: Investigation of the sensorimotor training using wireless sensor networks. Neurorehabilitation and neural repair **25**(9), 788–798 (2011)
13. Thiers, A., l'Orteye, A., Orlowski, K., Schrader, T.: *Analyse der muskulären Stabilisation während des sensomotorischen Trainings bei Verwendung von Geräten mit ein- und mehrdimensionaler Instabilität mit Hilfe von drahtlosen Sensoren.* GMDS 2013 58. Jahrestagung der Deutschen Gesellschaft für Medizinische Informatik, Biometrie und Epidemiologie (GMDS) e.V. (2013)
14. SENIAM project: Sensor Placement, http://www.seniam.org
15. Weineck, J.: Optimales Training. Spitta Verlag GmbH & Co, Balingen (2004)
16. Merletti, R., Parker, P.A.: Electromyography. Wiley, New Jersey (2004)
17. Gu, Y.D., Li, J.S., Ruan, G.Q., Wang, Y.C., Lake, M.J., Ren, X.J.: Lower limb muscles SEMG activity during high-heeled Latin dancing. In: Lim, C.T., Goh, J.C.H. (eds.) IFMBE Proceedings, vol. 31, pp. 198–200. SPringer, Heidelberg (2010)
18. Robertson, G., Caldwell, G., Hamill, J., Kamen, G., Whittlesey, S.: Research Methods in Biomechanics. Human Kinetics, Champaign (2004)
19. Medved, V.: Measurement of Human Locomotion. CRC Press, Boca Raton (2000)
20. Kaplanis, P.A., Pattichis, C.S., Hadjileontiadis, L.J., Roberts, V.C.: Surface EMG analysis on normal subjects based on isometric voluntary contraction. J. Electromyogr. Kinesiol. **19**(1), 157–171 (2009). Elseiver
21. Grimshaw, P., Lees, A., Fowler, N.: Sport and Exercise Biomechanics (BIOS Instant Notes). Bios Scientific Publisher, Abingdon (2006)
22. Lukas, C.M.: Kraftverhalten und elektromyographische Untersuchungen an der Unterschenkelmuskulatur bei Patienten nach operativ versorgter Achillessehnenruptur, http://www.drlukas.de/html/promotion.html

Scenarios for Sharing Good Practices
in Sport Management

André Boder[1]([⊠]), Christophe Barthe[2], and Antoine Sacoun[2]

[1] UEFA, Nyon, Switzerland
andre.boder@uefa.ch
[2] Metasud, London, England
{christophe,antoine}@metasud.com

Abstract. The European football governing body (UEFA) has developed a programme to share good practices in the management of sport. It includes blended learning (face-to-face and on-line interactive courses), knowledge sharing platforms and a 3D virtual stadium. The programme consists in collecting existing practices, creating new practices, organising them into an on-line platform and combining them into learning scenarios. Typical knowledge management issues are addressed such as integrating contextual and generic knowledge or yet turning tacit into explicit knowledge. The scenarios include libraries of good practices in the form of *learning objects* (videos and documents) as well as hints to solve critical problems in each of the domains of sport management.

Keywords: e-Learning · Best practices · Communities of practice · Information sharing · Learning organization · Organizational learning · Knowledge management · Sport management

1 Needs and Objectives

Over the past few years, the organisation of sport events and the administration of sport altogether have evolved tremendously. As a result a lot of good practices[1] have been created. But lessons learned are not applied systematically and good practices are often duplicated leading to a lack of professionalism and loss of efficiency. Indeed knowledge management has been advocated by various authors as a key aspect of the evolution of organisations [1–3].

One of the main reasons why good practices are not applied on a systematic basis is because they are not often made explicit. And the implementation of solutions also differs depending on the context of application. As a result, a number of attempts to address these issues have only been partly successful. Courses and workshops have not managed to really bring to bear the core of expertise required in the management of sport events for instance. There are two reasons for this. Firstly, the specific knowledge required in different contexts is not sufficiently distinguished from generic or standard

---

[1] The term « good practice » is used instead of « best practice », because practices may be more adequate than others depending on the context of application. Hence, there can be more than one unique best practice to address various situations.

© Springer International Publishing Switzerland 2015
J. Cabri et al. (Eds.): icSPORTS 2013, CCIS 464, pp. 72–84, 2015.
DOI: 10.1007/978-3-319-17548-5_6

knowledge. Secondly, the tacit knowledge of experts is not made explicit to a sufficient degree so as to allow practitioners to really grab the skills to master the processes involved [4]. In addition, learning scenarios lack interactivity. Hence, applications of good practices in particular cases, in-depth case studies, as well as answers to specific problems are not addressed to an extend that would allow practitioners to easily manage issues occurring in their own situations. When good practices are made explicit and when differentiation between various contexts of application have been taken into account, then new problems and new requirements turn up, leading to the creation of new practices in a never ending evolving process [5].

On top of these issues, a more practical issue hinders the sharing of good practices. It is often rather difficult to spot one's own problems and hence to search for adequate solutions. Therefore knowing how to make your problem explicit and knowing how to initiate your search for solutions is not obvious. This means that both the search devices and the organisation of the knowledge altogether need to be well thought out. But this is not obvious for the simple reason that knowledge is evolving, therefore requiring a constant update and a constant reorganisation of previous knowledge. In effect, addressing the need of a large community of practitioners and designing interactive environments in order to create contextual practices rather than only proposing a standard textbook calls for a system that is adaptive and evolving. Today, the technical tools exist to allow for just-in-time evolution of knowledge. The challenge is more one of design of the learning scenarios and a cultural one to get the buy-in of the various practitioners.

In order to respond to this need, the European football governing body (UEFA) has developed a programme to share good practices. The objective is to collect, create, organise and share the good practices across the football family (associations, confederations, clubs, coaches, referees, medical doctors etc.).

The programme's objectives include:

- The identification of existing opportunities as well as the design of new opportunities where good practices may be captured, shared and used. It can be either training sessions to prepare sport events, workshops to teach sport administrators, interviews of experts or else the events themselves where good practices are displayed. Topics include event management, marketing, communication, media & communication, safety & security, legal issues, sport medicine, governance and more.
- The development of a network of content experts and knowledge brokers who both validate and organise the know how captured and set up scenarios for further knowledge sharing and learning programmes.
- The design of learning objects which are the key components of the knowledge environment. They can be videos, on-line presentations, PDF documents, storytelling clips or yet structured courses in any domain of sport management. These learning objects originate in the various settings mentioned above. Namely, they can either consist of shots of real sport events, or else interviews of experts or yet reports or documents of any kind.
- The design of a series of scenarios to share knowledge, built from the combination of learning objects. The scenarios fall into two categories. Face-to-face and on-line.

Face-to-face scenarios include workshops, focused groups and simulations of sport management activities. On-line scenarios include the exhibition of multiple learning objects to browse from (with the possibility for the practitioner both to download and to upload new pieces of knowledge), a problem-solving oriented section to find ways to address specific issues and a series of e-learning structured courses that display standard knowledge in any domain of sport management. In some cases, the scenarios include certification programmes, diplomas as well as master's degree programmes. Besides their training objectives, these programmes serve as additional sources where knowledge can be captured and organized in the knowledge environment, therefore making them not only an educational tool but also a tool to develop and implement knowledge among a community of practitioners.

- The development of the knowledge environment itself consisting in various knowledge platforms including a knowledge interface named UEFA PLAY, an e-learning platform and a 3D interface.

2 Approach

The devices and functionalities of the knowledge environment have been designed on the basis of the status of the knowledge dealt with. Namely, good practices are pieces of knowledge that directly stem from the use and applications in the real world. The learning objects built from these pieces are not necessarily "validated knowledge". Hence, the status of these elements of knowledge is a heuristic one. They serve for the progressive construction of more standard knowledge which will crystallize after subsequent cross-fertilization through sharing and use in multiple contexts, which emphasizes the importance of sharing ideas in working communities [6].

On this basis, a number of orientations have been selected. For instance, the approach is clearly interactive, allowing for co-creation of knowledge in the context of sport events and training settings. It includes «shadowing sessions» whereby professionals follow experts in a particular task during a sport event. Similarly, it includes blended learning (including face-to-face and on-line interactive courses). One of the reason co-creation is a key parameter is because it induces comparisons between various practices, therefore generating a space for contextual practices, which depend on local specificities as well as for generic practices which cut across the different cultures [7].

Also, the knowledge sharing environment has been designed not only for browsing through a repository of items, but also to respond to the users' most common and most critical issues. It is problem solving oriented. For each topic, a set of answers is provided in the form of «how to», accompanied by a few hints to address a task coherently. These "how to" are updated as time flows by users who provide input to the knowledge base.

Because of the multipurpose nature of the programme (learning, knowledge sharing or yet problem solving), the knowledge sharing platform has been designed around three complementary concepts. One is modularity. Material is selected from a back-office knowledge repository and reorganized in various ways to shape the various scenarios. Then, the learning objects must be detailed enough so as to respond to the issues addressed. In other words, the granularity of the content must correspond to key aspects of the knowledge encapsulated in a module. Finally it is combinatorial, meaning the various elements can be aggregated to form higher-level elements to compose learning scenarios.

3 Implementation

In order to implement the approach described above, the model presented here in Fig. 1 displays the various steps of the knowledge management loop including creation, organisation, sharing and use of knowledge.

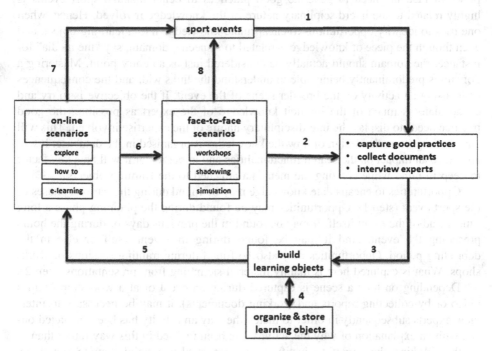

Fig. 1. The various steps of the knowledge management loop including creation, organisation, sharing and use of knowledge.

Steps 1 and 2 show how opportunities to create or collect knowledge are identified, from both the sport events themselves or else from training sessions (mainly workshops). Then after knowledge has been captured, learning objects are created in order to package the good practices into modular elements (step 3). Learning objects then need to be organized and classified (step 4). Three different types of scenarios for knowledge sharing are designed for on-line access on the platform (step 5). These scenarios may either be incorporated into face-to-face scenarios of knowledge sharing (step 6) or else put into application to be used in real life (step 7). Face-to-face scenario may also be put into application (step 8).

3.1   Capturing and Creating Good Practices

Sport events are complex because they include a mixture of different domains of sport management. And there is a need for coherence between the parts. Because the parts are interdependent, the analysis of skills required to manage an event and the good practices generated overtime are interdisciplinary. For instance, marketing operations during an event depend on the characteristics of a stadium which itself is linked with security and safety issues. In addition, management of the media is a key element since the major revenues are driven from broadcasting of the events.

This picture shows rather clearly that good practices are subtle pieces of knowledge and that they cannot be reduced to simple principles underlying each isolated discipline. In fact, the need to generate good practices to better manage sport events is highly related to the interdisciplinary nature of the knowledge involved. Hence, when one tries to identify opportunities to encapsulate knowledge into a learning object, and even though the piece of knowledge is related to a specific domain, say "the media" for instance, the domain should actually be considered just as an entry point. Mastering a domain is predominantly being able to understand the links with and the consequences of realising an activity on the broader scene of the event. If the objective is to try and encapsulate as much of the implicit knowledge of the expert as possible, the good practice needs to display the interdisciplinary nature of the expertise involved. This will have an impact on the design of how the knowledge is organised in the database. It will also have an impact on the search functionalities and in particular it will be a key factor to keep in mind while creating the metadata attached to the learning objects.

Opportunities to encapsulate knowledge may be found during the various phases of the sport event (step 1). Opportunities may be found during the planning phase a long time ahead of the event itself. It may be found in the previous days or during the hours preceding the event. And it may be found during the event itself or else in the debriefing period. Opportunities may also be found during training sessions or workshops. What is captured here is mainly material stemming from presentations (step 2).

Depending on how a scene is captured during an event or at a workshop (with a video or by collecting reports and working documents), it may be necessary to interview experts subsequently in order to match the way an activity has been managed on-site with an explanation of why the activity has been realised in this way rather than in another. Asking the expert to justify a practice is also a good way to pin down alternative actions which might have been less appropriate. This is also a way to refer to failures which are usually difficult to capture, since it is less likely the case that experts will agree to talk about them. One particular interesting way to capture knowledge is story-telling. Experts have been asked to tell stories and to make it explicit what the lessons learned are in each case. Actually, story-telling has proven so strong to encapsulate knowledge that it has been implemented into a specific type of learning object[2].

---

[2] A few more knowledge management techniques to capture knowledge have been used to build good practices. They are not presented here. They include observation, simulation, problem solving or yet comparison between practices.

3.2 Building Learning Objects

As online knowledge platforms are being used more and more in training and sharing knowledge and information, the amount of digital resources is beginning to increase and accumulate. Organisation and classification of these resources is becoming a major issue. For the reusability and interoperability, knowledge should be broken down into "chunks", (small pieces). They define the learning objects (step 3).

Among the many existing definitions of learning objects, IEEE's learning Technology Standards Committee proposed:

"Learning objects are defined here as any entity, digital or non-digital, which can be used, re-used or referenced during technology supported learning. Examples of technology supported learning include computer-based training systems, interactive learning environments, intelligent computer-aided instruction systems, distance learning systems, and collaborative learning environments."

The way we use digital resources in our project is close to the way Wiley defines the learning object as "any digital resource that can be re-used to support learning" [8]. This more precise definition is broad enough to include all available resources over a network (online), whether large or small, unique or consisting of a combination of different media.

Thus, the learning object built may be composed of "small digital resources" such as graphic images, videos, audio resources, portable document format (PDF), but also more complex ones, such as synchronized presentations texts and videos, interactive videos, or storytelling combining images, sounds, and interviews.

3.3 Organizing and Storing Learning Objects

Creating Metadata. Some information should be added to describe the learning object and to facilitate the search or the management of the learning object. This information is called metadata. Metadata helps make the resource searchable and reusable.

Metadata consists in descriptive information about digital resources including creation date, publishing date, title, author, description, keywords, photo, size, topics, location, etc. The metadata model must be standard. Hence, IEEE Standard for Learning Object Metadata (IEEE LOM) developed by IEEE LTSC (Learning Technology Standards Committee) has been used.

The content creator or administrator of the database provides metadata. The perception that metadata is complex and technical can be an issue for users. Local standards need to be defined and an easy and flexible tool needs to be provided to maintain the benefit of the metadata. The challenge is to understand how users will use metadata to search and classify information in order to simplify the tagging system and choose the most pertinent metadata fields for the main users.

Metadata is an essential element of the UEFA PLAY knowledge platform. Indeed, the classification of each learning object by topics, origin and date is necessary to enable the selection of resources through filters and tags and to use a full text search engine.

Learning Object Repository. Learning objects are stored in a database called Learning Object Repository. One of the key features of the repository is centralization. A wide variety of resources collected from multiple sources can thus be hosted in a central location. The repository works as a hub which provides a unique location to share digital resources for direct use or aggregation into scenarios (step 4).

In addition to providing access and centralized hosting, the repository allows administrators to authorize and control access to resources and hence protect the intellectual property rights of owners and creators.

The quality of learning objects is a key issue. To protect and maintain the integrity of information contained in the repository and to make sure that the users can acquire the right knowledge, experts are selected to take over responsibilities of specific domains. The guideline here is to ensure quality over quantity.

3.4   Designing On-Line Scenarios

The three knowledge sharing scenarios created in the platform (step 5) are based upon various ways to apprehend knowledge. One is open access and browsing. The second one is problem-solving and the third one is through material structured in more formal courses. Because the idea is to suggest to practitioners to build their own contextual practices, the best way to achieve this goal is to help them work both top down and bottom up. The formal courses provide them with ways to address the various aspects of a domain in a top down manner. Reciprocally, browsing through other material is a way to work bottom up and to grab new ideas. The problem solving scenario works both top down and bottom up. First it suggests a number of hints to tackle the problem in a systematic manner (top down). Also, it provides the practitioner with examples of ways in which a particular problem has been addressed by others (bottom up) (Fig. 2).

Exploring Knowledge. A number of functionalities have been included in the tag "EXPLORE". Firstly a filter allows selecting the year of production of the good practices. Secondly the origin of the good practice may be chosen. Thirdly, the domain it belongs to may also be selected. As for the origin of a learning object, it is not only interesting from the point of view of knowing its source. The main interest is to be able to compare practices which are contextual and respond to local needs, with more standard practices, such as those put into place by UEFA or academic partners for instance. This comparison helps practitioners carve their own practice both on the basis of other local solutions and also from good practices which have already been "validated" by the community to some degree.

Solving Problems. The tag "HOW TO" has been designed in order to help practitioners to address specific problems. The hints and examples are useful elements to carve their own solutions. In addition, the learning objects provided as examples display both the practices themselves and the reasons underlying the action. Hence, this is a way to turn tacit knowledge (lying in the expert's head) into explicit knowledge. This is particularly important because, as Sandberg has shown [9] different experts may have totally different mental models while achieving a task. Solving a specific problem and creating a

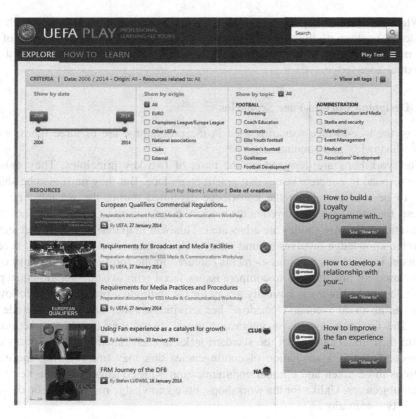

Fig. 2. The platform interface featuring three entry points, corresponding to various ways to apprehend knowledge (browsing, problem solving and structured learning), through the tags "explore", "how to" and "learn" (Source: UEFA PLAY platform, 2014).

contextual good practice depends highly on the possibility for the practitioner first to integrate and adapt an existing solution and second to understand the reasons why such a solution has been put in place. For this purpose, the environment includes a number of learning objects that display both aspects of the knowledge, such as the story-telling device where lessons learned from the story are made explicit by the expert.

e-Learning. Besides providing elements of knowledge to browse through, the platform includes a section (the tag "LEARN") where knowledge is structured and organised according to the standards in the various domains of sport management. The format chosen is interactive e-learning courses. The courses include formal presentations by top experts of the fields, as well as exercises and quiz to test the practitioners' skills. Because the e-learning sits on an LMS[3], it is possible to track the practitioner to help her on the different exercises. Tracking has also been used to assess practitioners in the scenarios where certificates were delivered.

---

[3] LMS: Learning Management System that follows the student involved in a learning process.

While this section displays more formatted and validated knowledge, each chapter includes a number of links to the learning objects found in other sections of the platform. This is an important aspect to facilitate the integration of standard and contextual knowledge.

3.5 Designing Face-to-Face Scenarios

Most of the face-to-face scenarios used in the programme are of three types: workshops, shadowing and simulations.

The workshops are designed on the basis of two key principles. They must of course respond to concrete issues that practitioners face. But they must also be shaped so as to be able to capture the knowledge exhibited during the sessions. For this purpose, the knowledge displayed in the workshop sessions must be modular, i.e., short presentations and case studies are advocated. This will help design learning objects in which the knowledge revolves around rather well focused issues. In addition, because the model is recursive, previous elements captured in the form of learning objects are usually used for practitioners to compare issues faced with existing solutions (step 6).

While the shadowing is basically a way for the individual practitioner to follow an expert during a real event and "shadow" her activities on-site, simulations include two parts. The first part consists in interactive visual discussions in which practitioners confirm their understanding of the standard tasks in each function of the sport event. The second part is a simulation of contingencies that may occur during the event. Decisions to be taken and optimal communication with colleagues are the key pedagogical objectives. Unlike for the workshops, little knowledge may usually be captured in these two scenarios.

3.6 Applying the Good Practices

The final goal in the whole process of capturing, creating, organising and sharing good practices is obviously to be able to apply them in the daily operations of managing sport activities (steps 7 & 8). In the programme, UEFA has put into place a number of local procedures to assist practitioners to implement lessons learned in the various knowledge sharing scenarios, such as focused groups, communities of practice, development of targeted projects or yet processes to cascade the knowledge more in-depth into local contexts.

4 Technology

4.1 Overview

The UEFA PLAY platform is linked to FAME which is the UEFA management application. FAME allows resources storage in various formats and the administration of user privileges.

UEFA PLAY offers intuitive filtering and search tools, in addition to semantic document grouping. To do this, UEFA PLAY links with the existing FAME database, creates its own learning repository and enriches resources with new properties (specific METADATA) not available in FAME.

4.2   Knowledge Platform Architecture

UEFA PLAY is a web application developed with the Symfony 2 PHP object oriented framework. It uses HTML 5/CSS 3/JavaScript (jQuery) standards. It has its own database based on MySQL programming language, which contains the properties added to the resources and the administrative privileges granted to users.

To operate robustly and to keep the concept of central database, UEFA PLAY has a replica of a subset of the data from the FAME database.

4.3   Data Replication from FAME to UEFA PLAY

Schematically, the exchange of data between FAME and UEFA PLAY works one way and uses XML files. This choice is mainly due to the different database technologies on both sides: SQL Server for FAME and MySQL for UEFA PLAY.

FAME Export. On FAME side, a subset of the data model has been previously defined. Only certain columns from some of the tables are considered. An application mechanism detects all changes made to data in the concerned subset (INSERT, UPDATE, DELETE) and publishes an XML file describing the change. The file is named with a unique ID based on the table, the key of the concerned row, the date and time to the nearest second. The publication is made on a shared FTP server (Fig. 3).

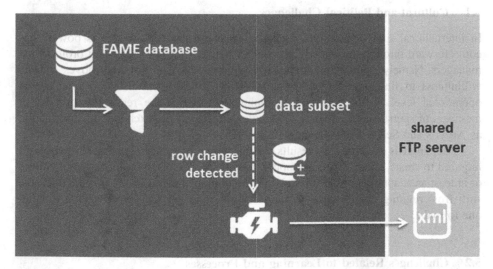

Fig. 3. The role of the FAME database in the exchanges of data with the UEFA PLAY platform.

UEFA PLAY Import. On its side, UEFA PLAY reads each incoming XML file and performs the required change on its FAME replica. Once treated, the XML file is moved to a different directory whether it triggered an error or not. Error detection is a key characteristic of the import mechanism. A specific chapter is dedicated to this. When an error is triggered, the application administrator is notified by email. Once investigation is made and the problem is found, failed files can be reprocessed by moving them back to the incoming directory.

The import mechanism is executed every 15 minutes thanks to an OS scheduling program. A script is called which performs a HTTP GET request on a specific URL, launching the import.

4.4   Authentication Through FAME

Since FAME is responsible for the confidentiality of the documents, the UEFA PLAY authentication mechanism is delegated to FAME.

Fame provides a login page dedicated to UEFA PLAY allowing to control which users can access the application. Furthermore, it allows single sign on between FAME and UEFA PLAY.

5   Challenges

Three types of challenges have been encountered in the course of the programme. Cultural & political challenges, challenges related to learning & processes and knowledge management challenges. Following are a few examples of these.

5.1   Cultural and Political Challenges

In international sport federations, the classical constraint "knowledge is power" has come forward through the underlying conflict between top hierarchy and professional managers. Namely, sport is predominantly governed through political moves and the willingness to link political strategies with the development of good practices at operational level is not necessarily omnipresent. Hence the reasoning process of members of sport federations may to some extent inhibit the exchange of information as Argyris and Schön have shown [10].

Also, sport is governed by results. In this frame of mind, focusing on *processes* required to create, adapt, share and apply new practices calls upon a change of culture or at least an adaptation of the roles assigned within the federation. More generally, the shift from running day-to-day *operations* to investing into *development* is a difficult one to make.

5.2   Challenges Related to Learning and Processes

When development has been accepted as a critical strategy, then another step has yet to be overcome. New methodologies based upon interactivity, knowledge sharing and with the support of technology must be accepted.

Another common challenge to face is to move away from the idea that a knowledge environment should provide ready-made solutions. Grabbing a few hints here and there, customizing them to your own context and carving your own good practices is not necessarily obvious for everyone.

5.3 Knowledge Management Challenges

You never start from scratch. Therefore, linking new practices to your own way of doing things is a challenge, not mentioning the technical challenge you face when you already have databases that need to become evolving databases if they were not designed with such a philosophy.

The level of granularity of knowledge is certainly the hardest challenge, since the usefulness of good practices strictly depends upon its applicability to as many situations you face as possible. If the learning objects are too detailed, they will not serve much of a purpose. On the contrary, if they are too general, they will not be seen as bringing an added value to the situation.

The issue of validation of knowledge is also a tricky one although in principle the idea behind the development of good practices is not to come up with a validating process in the same way as you would for scientific papers for instance. The term *good practice* is carved precisely to suggest that, depending on the context, a practice may be more adequate than another one. However, some practices are *standard* and therefore need to be progressively validated as "best practices", while others are not.

Finally, the biggest challenge probably stems from a huge confusion overwhelmingly present between document management and knowledge management. The paradigm behind the environment developed here is the recursive loop between the capture, organisation and reuse of good practices in the form of yet new sharing scenarios. The added value in the knowledge management process does not stem from just a one-time capture of knowledge and its storing into a database but precisely its progressive refinement through a recursive process [11].

6 Conclusion

Even though the platform appears as the key feature in the programme, it should not only be considered as a repository of knowledge, but rather as the result of a dynamic process of knowledge creation. Indeed, knowledge is created from subsequent applications of pre-existing elements of knowledge in different contexts, shared ideas in workshop sessions as well as interviews of experts leading to a constant updating of the content. Hence, every aspect of the development and evolution of knowledge is present through the programme. The result of this recursive loop is displayed in the form of learning objects called "good practices". Good practices can be considered as an intermediary phase in the progressive scientific construction of knowledge. It is a phase in which knowledge is extracted from reality but not yet confronted with a set of rigorous methodologies which will eventually turn them into scientifically validated knowledge. This phase can be considered as a breeding ground allowing for a constant generation of new pieces of knowledge.

The design of such an environment must obviously be based upon a careful analysis of users' needs and requirements. The platform emphasizes concrete hints, allowing for quick and easy solutions for the user. But at the same time, the idea is to trigger thinking and to induce comparisons between the various practices. Hence, the structure and the material have been conceived to provide both ready-made solutions but also to push the user to create his or her solution adapted to the specific context. This calls for an environment featuring a variety of ideas to choose from rather than rigid best practices.

The most critical requirement for the platform is clearly the user friendliness and the relevance and speed of results of the search function. Here, the platform's efficiency is dependent upon the way the metadata have been built in. Namely, the material shall not be tagged too narrowly, again allowing the user to compare between sometimes even contradictory possibilities to address a challenge.

References

1. Davenport, T.H., Prusak, L.: Working Knowledge. How Organizations Manage What They Know. Harvard Business School Press, Boston (1998)
2. Teece, D.J.: Managing Intellectual Capital. Oxford University Press, Oxford (2000)
3. Von Krogh, G., Roos, J., Kleine, D. (eds.): Knowing in Firms: Understanding, Managing and Measuring Knowledge. Sage, London (1998)
4. Sternberg, R.J., Horvath, J.A. (eds.): Tacit Knowledge in Professional Practice. Lawrence Erlbaum, Mahwah (1999)
5. Von Krogh, G., Ichijo, K., Nonaka, I.: Enabling Knowledge Creation. Oxford University Press, Oxford (2000)
6. Boder, A.: Collective intelligence: a keystone in knowledge management. J. Knowl. Manage. 10(1), 81–93 (2006)
7. Boder, A., Cavallo, D.: An epistemological approach to intelligent tutoring systems. Intell. Tutoring Media 1(1), 23–29 (1990)
8. Wiley, D.A.: Connecting learning objects to instructional design theory: a definition, a metaphor, and a taxonomy. In: Wiley, D.A. (ed.) The Instructional Use of Learning Objects. Association for Educational Communications and Technology, Bloomington (2000)
9. Sandberg, J.: Human Competence at Work. An Interpretative Approach. BAS, Göteborg (1994)
10. Argyris, C., Schön, D.: Organisational Learning: A Theory of Action Perspective. Addison-Wesley, Reading (1978)
11. Boder, A.: The process of reification in human-human interaction. J. Comput. Assist. Learn. 8(3), 177–185 (1992)

Application of Mobile Technologies
in the Preparations for Long Distance Running

Ladislav Havaš[1], Vladimir Medved[2(✉)], and Zoran Skočir[3]

[1] Department of Electrical Engineering, Polytechnic of Varaždin,
Križanićeva 33, Varaždin, Croatia
ladislav.havas@velv.hr
[2] Faculty of Kinesiology, University of Zagreb, Zagreb, Croatia
vladimir.medved@kif.hr
[3] Faculty of Electrical Engineering and Computing, University of Zagreb,
Zagreb, Croatia
zoran.skocir@fer.hr

Abstract. Fast development of mobile ICT technologies enabled and imposed their implementation in business and sports. As mobile technologies enable quick two-way communication, independent of the present location of athletes, their trainer or expert hardware and software systems, it is significantly important to utilize the advantages of that kind of communication to maximize the chances of achieving excellent results in a specific training process. This paper shows one ORT (Online Running Trainer) system, which was developed for preparations of marathon runners. It describes algorithms for calculation of training equivalents of set and achieved trainings, which was used for the success analysis of every micro cycle of the training process. By using available telecommunication channels, ORT system communicates with users in real time. It analyses their performance and, if necessary, dynamically corrects their training parameters to achieve better results in needed moment. Described methods are verified on a selected sample of runners.

Keywords: Expert system · Long distance running · Mobile ICT technologies · ORT · Training equivalent · Training process

1 Introduction

Nowadays, modern mobile ICT technologies follow up an athlete in all stages of their preparations. It helps him in developing a program of their preparations, ensures him an access to important information in the right moment and enables the storage of current parameters and information related to training process or to a particular training. Major expansion in the development of mobile phones of all sizes, with great processing capabilities, affordable prices and intuitive user interface, has made the users of all sport, psychological and cognitive categories capable of using telecommunication services during the indoor and outdoor workouts. In that way, there are possibilities of an individual approach to a single athlete, regardless of their current location, and the communication between the athlete and their coach or between the athlete and the system that cares for athlete's results is facilitated. In a situation where there is an

© Springer International Publishing Switzerland 2015
J. Cabri et al. (Eds.): icSPORTS 2013, CCIS 464, pp. 85–99, 2015.
DOI: 10.1007/978-3-319-17548-5_7

expert system that has the ability to generate a program for athletic preparations and the ability to evaluate given and performed trainings in real time, mobile telecommunication channels become dominant communication platform between the system, a coach and his athlete.

In this paper is shown one such system which helps long-distance runners in developing their program for preparations, and by using available mobile ICT technologies it stores, analyzes the information and advices them in real or near-real time. Ineffective trainings are dynamically changed with solutions that are safer and that faster lead to the preferred result, with lesser chance of sport injury. The second part of this paper describes the architecture of one "Online running training system" (ORT), while the third part of the paper shows telecommunication platform which is used for two-way communication with users. The fourth part of the paper describes the methods and algorithms developed for evaluation of given and performed workouts in the preparation program for 5K runners to marathon runners. In the fifth part is described and shown the verification of results on a selected sample of marathon runners. The final part of the paper gives a conclusion and the list of references.

2   Representation of ORT System

The prototype of the system was developed by using open-source programs (PHP, MySQL, Linux). The whole applicative solution was launched on the Linux distribution of CentOS 6.4, version 5.3.3 of objectively-oriented PHP language, on MySQL server relational database distribution 5.67 [1], and on Apache web server 2.2.15. Individual applications are run by cron (crontab, cron table) service.

2.1   The Architecture of an Expert System

The first display which users of prototype of ORT system encounter is shown in the Fig. 1.

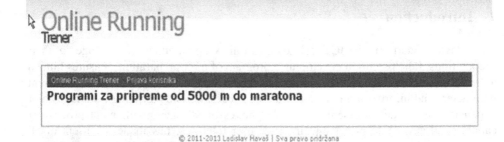

Programi za pripreme od 5000 m do maratona

© 2011-2013 Ladislav Havaš | Sva prava pridržana

Fig. 1. Opening display of prototype of ORT system (in Croatian language).

During the registration process, users define their user name and their password, they enter their personal info, the number of their mobile phone and their e-mail address where they receive an activation link. Due to the security reasons, user's password is encrypted with MD5 algorithm, 128-byte cryptography hash function, ratified Internet standard RFC 1321, and in that form it is being stored in the database. When the user has successfully logged in, he or she is presented with an appropriate menu, in accordance with his or her authorization levels. A specific part of the menu functions/options is shown or hidden from the user.

2.2 Generating the Training Program

One of the frequently used functions of the system is "Program generating". The main task of that subsystem is to create a program for preparations of long-distance runners for following distances:

- 5000 m (5K)
- 10000 m (10K)
- 21097 m (half marathon)
- 42195 m (marathon)

After the user enters the results of his/her current sport capabilities (race or training), the system calculates their maximum aerobic capacity ($VO2_{max}$ factor), which serves the purpose of estimating runner's potential on the races from 800 m to marathon, which is going to be used in the future workouts. Then the runner selects a specific discipline for which he intends to prepare, the length of the program (between 12 and 24 weeks), the starting date, selects the upper limit of the acceptable weekly mileage and decides on the toughness of the program (Program A – beginners), (Program B – advanced) or (Program C – elite). The opening display for entering the parameters needed for generating the program is shown in the Fig. 2.

2.3 Running Log

All the done workouts the user can and should inscribe in the second important module called the "Running Log" by using the available telecommunication channels and by doing so enable evaluation and the comparison of envisaged and performed workouts.

Selecting the appropriate day and the input of relevant data is possible to render in real time, during the workout or immediately after the workout, but also backwards, which allows the user to completely fill in the Running Log in order to get the review of your performance as detailed as possible. Aside from the usual track of each workout (when, how much, how fast, the type of training...), the user has the ability to mark their own training based on their biased perception (tiredness, lack of sleep, humidity, temperature, wind and other aggravating factors) through VAS scale (Visual Analog Scale), which is known as a frequently used medical psychometric method that has been used for evaluating the sense of pain. That scale enables the choice of values between 0 and 10, wherein 0 would stand for ideal conditions for a workout and values closer to 10 would stand for less ideal conditions, thereby done workouts should be

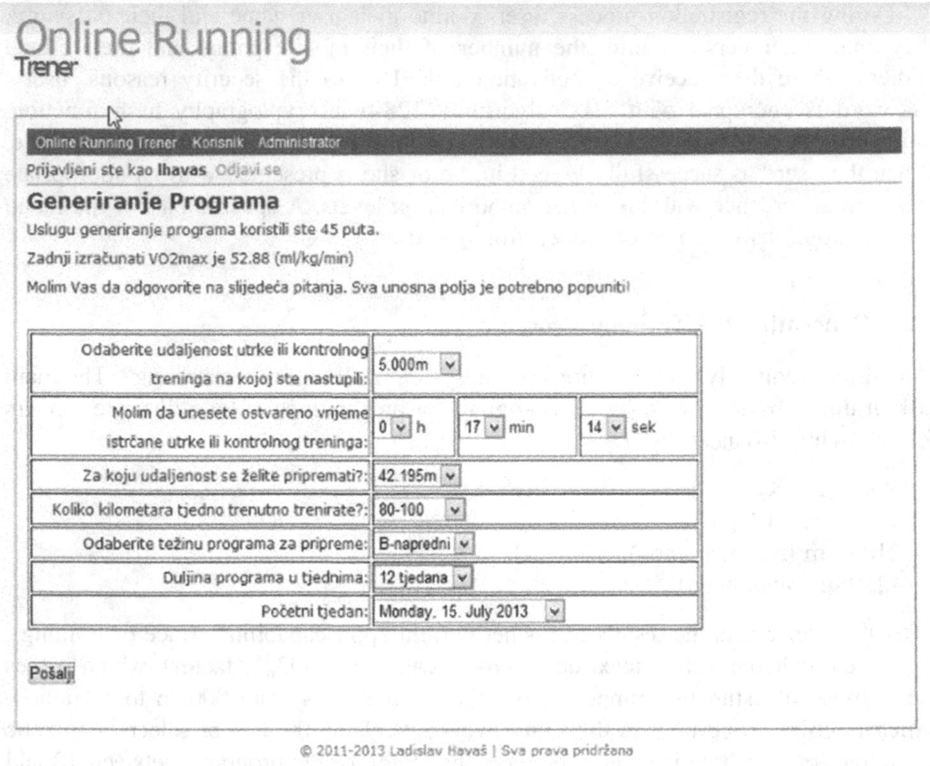

Fig. 2. Entering the basic parameters for generating the program (in Croatian language).

also assessed in accordance with appropriate correction factor. With the possibility of inputting the data through web (version 2.0), other methods have also been developed which use mobile telecommunication channels and allow the user to communicate with ORT system in real or almost real time through e-mail (smart phones) or through SMS.

3   The Architecture of the Telecommunication Platform

A telecommunication system was developed which has the purpose of enabling the exchange of information in real time with the users through several different telecommunication interfaces.

The information which the users exchange with ORT system have to be in a specific format which is set by the protocol for exchange of the data that is to be mentioned in the following parts of this paper. All information which, through different mobile channels, arrive to the system are being stored in the Running Log. From there they are periodically filling by ETL process (Extracting, Transforming, Loading) into the data warehouse, and after extensive analyzes users can inform themselves about the quality of their workouts in the past period of time. The flow of information between the user and the system is shown in the Fig. 3.

From the Fig. 3 can be seen that there are supported following methods for exchange of data between the user and the database:

- Web
- E-mail
- SMS

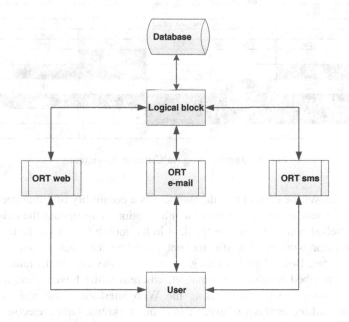

Fig. 3. The flow of information between the modules of the system.

By using different Internet browsers (Firefox, Google Chrome, Opera, Safari…) users inscribe their done workouts into the system, for the purpose of their use in the feedback analysis. In case of the e-mail method the users use available e-mail clients, which they sent their e-mail messages to. The advantage of this method lies in the fact that the majority of smart phones support e-mail function through some of available e-mail clients. In that way an interaction between distant users and the ORT system is enabled, provided that on a particular location there is a signal of one mobile network. SMS, as a third method for exchanging the information, enables the communication in real time with the users that are owners of older cell phones which do not possess an e-mail function. The limit of this communication method lies in the fact that the upper limit of characters in one sms is 160. In the follow-up, mentioned methods will be thoroughly presented.

3.1   ORT Web Module

By using the Web module, it is possible in a simple and intuitive way to develop a communication with a Running Log. By launching one of available Internet browsers and by entering the appropriate menu of ORT web application, one is able to update the Running Log. In the Fig. 4 it can be seen the opening display which a user sees upon entering.

Online Running Trener	Korisnik	Administrator				
Prijavljeni ste kao **lhavas** Odjavi se						

DAN Planirani trening		DAN Upisani trening		DAN Trening nije zadan		

Veljaca 2013						
<<	<		==		>	>>
Pon	Uto	Sri	Cet	Pet	Sub	Ned
				1	2	3
4	5	6	7	8	9	10
11	12	13	14	15	16	17
18	19	20	21	22	23	24
25	26	27	28			

Fig. 4. Running Log (in Croatian language).

It always shows the current month, but there is a possibility of going backwards, in case a runner wants to inscribe some new information or to update the existing ones.

Boxes labelled with red stand for the days in the month for which the user has been given a particular workout, but still has not inscribed feedback information on that particular workout. Boxes labelled with green stand for the days in the month for which the user has inscribed feedback information, whereas white boxes stand for the days when there is no given workout. Using the Web interface is the main method for determination and the analysis of given and done workouts. Other telecommunication channels such as e-mail and SMS are used in order to provide the runners with the ability to directly communicate with the application during or immediately after the workout.

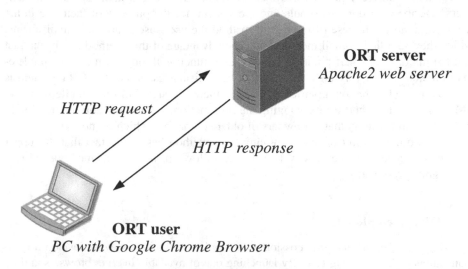

Fig. 5. HTTP transaction.

Access to the Web interface is enabled through HTTP protocol (Hypertext Transfer Protocol). HTTP protocol is the protocol of application (seventh) layer of OSI model (Open Systems Interconnection) and functions by using "Request-Response" method in which the Web server and the client participate.

On a server which runs ORT application is installed and set Apache2 Web server. That Web server is always active and awaits new requests on a network port 80. Upon receiving new HTTP request which is initiated by a client, i.e. user of a Web browser, web service will, from local disc, reach predefined data files inscribed in the form of HTML (HyperText Markup Language) record which presents ORT Running Log.

One such transaction is shown in the Fig. 5. This type of joining the database is impractical for mobile phones with small displays.

3.2 ORT e-Mail Module

This module is used for processing and sending e-mail messages. For its work it uses IMAP (Internet Message Access Protocol) and SMTP (Simple Mail Transfer Protocol) protocols. Module is, at very high frequency and through IMAP protocol, connects to a mailbox of an electronic mail of ORT system in which it finds e-mail messages of the users. The system will, in accordance with programmed protocol for exchanging the information, check the accuracy of information and will notify the user on the outcome of his request through SMTP protocol.

An example of the transaction performed through ORT e-mail module:

User inquiry:

```
From: lhavas@velv.hr
To: ort.trener@gmail.com
Subject: ?
```

A response from ORT system:

```
From: ort.trener@gmail.com
To: lhavas@velv.hr
Subject: ORT Help
Dear user,
Welcome to ORT system for training login through e-mail. In
order to receive help for a specific type of training please
enter one of the following phrases in the SUBJECT of an e-mail
message on the address ort.trener@gmail.com:
I? - for an interval training
S? - for a superset training
T? - for a tempo training
L? - for a prolonged training
R? - for a recovery training
X? - for an alternative training
Example: Subject: I?
Kind regards,
Your ORT!
```

In case the user, for example has done an interval training according to given instructions, it is possible to inscribe the training in the database through an e-mail in the following way:

```
From: lhavas@velv.hr
To: ort.trener@gmail.com
Subject:
#I*400*00:01:30*10*120*12000*60*180*120*145*980**7*demo
training example#
```

All successfully registered trainings are inscribed in the database in real time in the Running Log.

The next example shows an e-mail communication between the user and the ORT system in details:

An e-mail client, which is installed on the user's cell phone will connect, through SMTP protocol, with one of the outgoing e-mail servers and issue a request for sending an e-mail message of the predefined content. That e-mail server will parse an e-mail address on local-name@domein and will, based on that, draw a conclusion in which domain the user is located. Through DNS (Domain Name System) request, it will ask for MX (Mail Exchanger) record of the domain, whose response will provide it with the information on the list of names of serves and associated priorities for the domain in concern. E-mail server with the lowest priority will be the destination on which prior listed e-mail servers will send message to. When that message is being delivered to the destination server, it will be reachable in the user's mail box IMAP protocol, which is shown in the Fig. 6.

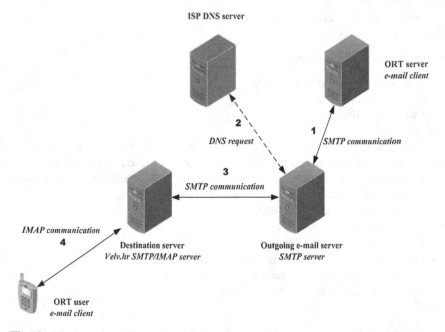

Fig. 6. Display of e-mail communication between the ORT server and the ORT user.

3.3   ORT SMS Module

The ORT *SMS module* is used for communication with the users whose mobile phones do not support e-mail function. With the fact that one sms is limited to 160 characters, the main flaw of this subsystem is in its unprofitability in regard to free and as fast e-mail messages. ORT system sends SMS messages by using SMS service called *Clickatell.com*.

Clickatell.com SMS service accepts HTTP request whose URL (Uniform Resource Locator) address possesses all needed information for sending SMS. As a HTTP response on the previous HTTP request, one receives a confirmation whether a message has been successfully sent. When Clickatell.com through HTTP protocol takes over all necessary information, SMS is, in accordance with the request, directed all the way to the tele-communication mobile operator on which there is a mobile phone of the ORT user.

4   Evaluation of the Training Quality

Dynamic management of training process is impossible without methods and algorithms for evaluation of the quality of given and performed workouts. The following segments of this paper will briefly describe the methods for calculating the numeric equivalent of basic training elements in the athletic preparations of marathon runners. Firstly, an algorithm for determining the training equivalent of given trainings will be described, then the procedure for evaluation of done training will be described.

4.1   Given Trainings

Long Run:

Long Run is the basis of all programs for long-distance running, and especially of the program for preparation of marathon runners [2]. The effort should not be too high as one should run in the aerobic zone.

Due to the above-mentioned reasons, for each 15 min of running, ORT system adds 5 points to the total training equivalent.

Tempo training:

During the determination of training equivalent in tempo training, potential of the user is also taken into consideration along with the duration of the training, in regard to his currently calculated maximal aerobic capacity $VO2_{max}$.

In case that a tempo training means running in the tempo of a marathon, the duration is calculated in seconds and compared with the anticipated capabilities of that particular runner. Calculated training equivalent is a percent of the training duration in seconds in regard to maximum duration in seconds which is anticipated for a user based on his anticipated result. Anticipating the potential is realized by a method of dr. Daniels and Gilbert [3].

Speed training:

From many known speed trainings, in ORT system are used Interval training and

Super set training.

The first step is to calculate the percentage of the run distance at the given tempo. In case one runs at the tempo of 5000 m race, and one runs 4000 m (10 × 400 m), that implies training equivalent of 80 %, or 80. That equivalent is decreased 0,5 points for every 15-s break between intervals.

Recovery training:

Recovery trainings are not physiologically demanding, which means that during the calculation of the training equivalent only the duration in the 15-min intervals is calculated. Every hour of such training gives the runner 20 points to the total training equivalent.

4.2 The Analysis of Done Trainings

When the database receives the data from done trainings, it is also necessary to calculate their training equivalent. Methods that are explained for calculating the training equivalent are used, although some new parameters are also introduced, for the purpose of even more detailed evaluation of achieved effects.

Aside from all known parameters that are used in trainings and serve the purpose of calculating the training equivalent (speed, duration, distance, number of trials, duration of recovery periods etc.), the user has the ability to inscribe some additional values:

- HR – maximum, minimum or average heart rate during the training
- Kcal – burned calories during the training
- Lactates – concentration of the lactic acid in the blood
- VAS - subjective estimate of the training conditions (temperature, humidity, wind, biorhythm, tiredness, lack of energy…)

Every one of those parameters influences the quality of the evaluation of done trainings.

HR (Heart Rate):

Each user should (by using some of the suggested methods [4] calculate their maximum heart rate and inscribe the data into the ORT system. By knowing the maximum heart rate of every user (HR_{max}), it is possible to estimate has the particular user resided in a specific HR zone, which is usual for that type of training.

Particular trainings and running tempos of a certain part should be done within one of the zones [5]:

- Zone 1: 50−60 % of the maximum heart rate (very easy, daily activities)
- Zone 2: 60–70 % of the maximum heart rate (easy activity, fat burning zone)
- Zone 3: 70–80 % of the maximum heart rate (aerobic zone, a moderate effort)
- Zone 4: 80–90 % of the maximum heart rate (anaerobic threshold)
- Zone 5: 90–100 % of the maximum heart rate (very intense, competitive training)

In case a particular type of training is done within the appropriate zone, it is not necessary to correct the calculated training equivalent. For every jump to a lower or to a higher zone, the system calculates ± 20 points to the training equivalent.

Calories (Kcal):

There is no exact method which would allow for a precise calculation of how many calories a runner of a certain weight, sex and years of age consumes at a certain speed of running in a particular period of time or a duration interval. On top of that, it has been noticed that there is a specific correlation between the heart rate and the consumption of calories for user. One of the more quality methods that takes into account above-mentioned parameters as well as maximum aerobic capacity has been suggested in [6] and it was used in the prototype of the ORT system for calculating the number of consumed calories. In case where the maximum aerobic capacity $VO2_{max}$ of an individual is known, then:

formula for men is:

$$((-95.7735 + (0.634 \times HR) + (0.404 \times VO2_{max}) + (0.394 \times W) + (0.271 \times A))/4.184)$$
$$\times 60 \times T$$

$$(1)$$

formula for women is:

$$((-59.3954 + (0.45 \times HR) + (0.380 \times VO2max) + (0.103 \times W) + (0.274 \times A))/4.184)$$
$$\times 60 \times T$$

$$(2)$$

Where is:

HR = heart rate per minute
W = weight in kilograms
A = age in years
T = duration in hours
$VO2_{max}$ = max. aerobic capacity in ml/kg/min

Lactates:

The speed of creating lactic acid is proportional to the speed of running, i.e. it is proportional to the percentage of used maximum aerobic capacity. For the trainings that are at marathon tempo, the concentration of the lactic acid should not be crossing the level of 2 mmol/L of blood. For the runs that are at the tempo of half-marathon, it is predicted that lactates do not cross the level of 4 mmol/L of blood, while for the runs at the tempo of races on 10000, 5000 and 3000 m, the concentration of the lactic acid is significantly higher than 4 mmol/L of blood. Every discrepancy from the prescribed intervals, the ORT system evaluates with the correction of the training equivalent by ± 15 points.

VAS (Visual Analogue Scale):

In the ORT system it is used as a unique indicator of the quality of the training conditions. For all values between 0–4 it is considered that the conditions were adequate, and accordingly the training effect remains unchanged. For each value higher than 4, calculated training effect is increased by 5 points.

Mentioned values can be subjected to certain changes for the purpose of increasing the quality of training evaluation. Since the developed system has the ability of self-learning, those parameters will be changed in time to more optimal values of those factors.

5 Verification and Analysis of the Results

5.1 Verification of the Results

Developed system for generating programs and the mobile surveillance of the quality of the training process has been verified on a selected sample of marathon runners, which allowed for an evaluation of the quality of implemented methods and algorithms, for the purpose of correcting or updating, if necessary, some of the methods used. Selected and analyzed were the runners of both sexes and in the age range from 18 to 65.

The number of people who have fulfilled all of the above-mentioned conditions is 58. Among that group there were some beginners, some advanced runners and some were the elite runners who have won many marathons and ultra marathons.

In the Table 1 is shown one part of the users who have participated in the process of the results verification. For the sake of easier statistical analysis, all time measures into seconds.

Table 1. Display of one part of verified users and their results.

No.	Sex	Year of birth	VO2max (ml/kg/min)	Planned result (s)	Achieved result (s)
1	male	1966.	59,32	2:49:00 (10140)	2:55:21 (10521)
2	male	1987.	33,48	4:28:00 (16080)	4:31:22 (16282)
3	male	1970.	56,32	2:55:00 (10500)	3:02:12 (10932)
4	male	1994.	43,12	3:40:00 (13200)	3:38:19 (13099)
5	male	1983.	30,82	4:45:00 (17100)	4:52:11 (17531)
6	female	1982.	50,52	3:09:00 (11340)	3:07:20 (11240)
7	male	1978.	49,22	3:10:00 (11400)	3:08:40 (11320)

5.2 Statistical Analysis of the Results

IAAF (International Association of Athletics Federations) evaluates runners and their results in 5-year classes, and in this paper the runners and their results are evaluated according to their sex and whether they are between 18–29, 30–50 and more than 50 years of age. Moreover, they have also been assessed according to toughness level of their preparations. Program A (marathon slower than 3:30:00), Program B (marathon between 3:00:00 and 3:30:00) and Program C (marathon faster than 3:00:00).

For the analysis of included data, a descriptive statistical analysis was used [7], while for the graphical display of data distribution there were used rectangular diagrams (Box and Whisker plot). Statistical processing of data has been done by using a mathematical applicative programme "Matlab 7.0.1" and the application Microsoft Excel 2013. Statistically significant in the analysis were confirmed discrepancies at the significance level of $p < 0,01$.

Athletes included in the research were old, on average, 34,16 years, wherein the standard deviation is 9,87 years. Range of variation has the value of 47 since the youngest participant is 18, while the oldest is 65.

During the research of correlation between achieved and planned result, Pearson's coefficient of correlation has been calculated. Based on the value of the coefficient of correlation and the p-value derived during the testing of the hypothesis on statistical significance of the analyzed variables ($r = 0,9926$ and $p = 0,0000$), it can be concluded that there is a statistically significant positive correlation between the observed variables. The graphical display of the correlation between achieved and planned result is given in the Fig. 7.

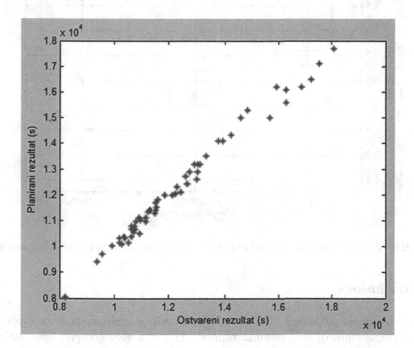

Fig. 7. Correlation between achieved and planned result (in Croatian language).

Distribution of the data obtained during the research has been verified with "Kolmogorov – Smirinov" test. Since the distribution of the data substantially deviates from the normal distribution, for calculating statistically significant discrepancies between the three groups has been used non-parameter (Kruskal-Wallis) test. The results of the Kruskal-Wallis test, which relate to planned time for the programs A, B and C indicates that there is statistically significant difference in planned time between the groups ($H = 50,4978$ and $p = 0,0000$). Test for multiple comparison has confirmed that all three groups (three toughness levels) are statistically substantially different. In order to achieve that kind of results, in more than 50 % of the users it was necessary to dynamically modify the training process.

Figure 8 gives a graphical display of the drawn conclusion from a statistical test.

All necessary corrections of implemented algorithms and the evaluation of particular training elements were automatically implemented into the system.

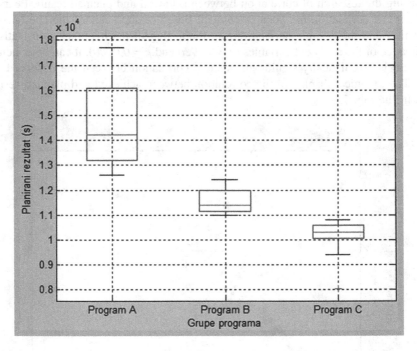

Fig. 8. Planned result (s) in regard to different toughness level (in Croatian language).

6 Conclusions

This paper shows modelling of a system for mobile telecommunication support in athletic preparations of long-distance runners. This is a very complex area which is intensively growing and in the future is going to be a subject of many analyzes and the opportunity for implementation of new ideas and algorithms.

Here was described one telecommunication platform which in real time communicates with athletes, evaluates their given and done workouts, and, if necessary, dynamically modifies the rest of their training process for the purpose of achieving better results. Functioning of an expert system which generates programs for preparations in popular long-distance disciplines (5000 m, 10000 m, half-marathon and marathon) was presented in this paper. Developed system is dimensioned for simultaneous interactive use by a large group of users. Flexible environment was created which protects the individuality of each athlete, who decides on their own on the volume of their training, the starting date, toughness level as well as chooses one of the available telecommunication channels for the data transfer. As opposed to many other web services and available books, at this point there it does not end the interaction with the developed system. Database and the data warehouse were formed which are being updated in real time and the algorithms for evaluation of given and done trainings have also been developed.

Research on this topic has been directed at integration of all above-mentioned segments, generated program and the feedback information in the shared database, by using mobile telecommunication channels for data transfer in real or almost-real time. Verification of the algorithms and the methods has been conducted on a limited sample of marathon runners. The procedure of verification where the database and the data warehouse have been filled with new quality data on daily basis has led to enabled self-learning and constant improvement of implemented algorithms for generating programs for evaluation of results.

By a modular concept of the database the data warehouse and by using the technologies and the tools of open-source codes, it is relatively easy to extend the system with new hardware and software modules.

The procedure of verification has shown that dynamic correction of generated programs in real time, by using ICT technologies and implemented algorithms and methods, substantially decreases the probability of not achieving adequate result with the increased probability of achieving the desired result in optimal conditions.

References

1. MySQL (2013). http://www.mysql.com/. Accessed 07 July 2013
2. Havaš, L., Vlahek, P.: Road running (in Croatian). TK Međimurje, Čakovec (2006)
3. Daniels, J.T., Gilbert, J.: Oxygen Power: Performance Tables for Distance Runners. Oxygen Power, Tempe (1979)
4. Heart rate training zones (2013). http://www.brianmac.co.uk. Accessed 01 Apr 2013
5. Polar sport zones for running (2012). http://www.polar.com/en. Accessed 29 Dec 2012
6. Keytel, L.R., Goedecke, J.H., Noakes, T.D., Hiiloskorpi, H., Laukkanen, R., van der Merwe, L., Lambert, E.V.: Prediction of energy expenditure from heart rate monitoring during sub-maximal exercise. J. Sports Sci. **23**(3), 289–297 (2005)
7. Lipschutz, S., Schiller, J.: Schaum's Outline of Introduction to Probability and Statistics. McGraw-Hill, New York (1998)

Author Index

Printed in the United States
By Bookmasters